101 Things to Do Before You Diet

101 Things to Do Before You Diet

Because Looking Great Isn't Just About Losing Weight

MIMI SPENCER

RODALE

Rodale books may be purchased for business or promotional use or for special sales. For information, please write to: Special Markets Department, Rodale Inc., 733 Third Avenue, New York, NY 10017

Printed in the United States of America
Rodale Inc. makes every effort to use acid-free ∞, recycled paper ♻.

Book design by Tara Long
Illustrations by Brandi Powell/istock

Library of Congress Cataloging-in-Publication Data
Spencer, Mimi.
   101 things to do before you diet : because looking great isn't just about losing weight / Mimi Spencer.
      p.   cm.
   Includes index.
   ISBN-13 978–1–60529–848–1 hardcover
   ISBN-10 1–60529–848–4 hardcover
   1. Beauty, Personal. 2. Dinners and dining. I. Title. II. Title: One hundred one things to do before you diet.
   HQ1219.S74 2009
   646.7'042—dc22
                                            2009014759

Distributed to the trade by Macmillan
2   4   6   8   10 9 7 5 3 1   hardcover

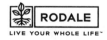

We inspire and enable people to improve their lives and the world around them

For more of our products visit **rodalestore.com** or call 800-848-4735

For Lily and Ned

CONTENTS

CH 3   BODY BASICS: IT STARTS IN YOUR PANTS   48

CH 4   HOW TO EAT PETITE, PART I: WHAT TO PUT ON YOUR FORK   65

INTRODUCTION

THIN: THE DREAM OF A GENERATION

I don't know a woman who wouldn't like to lose a few pounds. Some, of course, would dearly love to lose more—a dress size or two—but most of us gaze mistily into the middle distance of our lives and envision a time when we'll be, oh, 7 pounds lighter, a time when a size-12 skirt doesn't pinch after lunch, when our jeans won't clutch at our thighs like a petulant toddler, when our stomach is more buff than muffin. For most of us, it's an irritating, persistent hum in the back rooms of our minds.

I'm not about to tell you to stop aspiring to be that little bit slimmer. As a 40-year-old woman with a healthy interest in looking fabulous in a clingy top, I recognize the desire that burns within all of us to make the very best of what we've got. I'm well aware of the female need to compete with her peers—how we all look at the bikini bodies on the beach to gauge whether we measure up, how bloody brilliant it feels to walk into a crowded room and know that people are sizing up the wiggle in your walk and not the wobble in your chin. Really, who doesn't want to look better, feel happier, and be fitter? We want to be in control of our lives. We want our appearance to reflect our aspirations—for our careers, for our children, for our sense of self. In short, and given the choice, most of us don't want to be fat.

This book is the simple, sign-posted route to achieving that goal. It describes exactly how you can arrive at a whole new you, a place where you'll feel, look, and *be* better than you ever have before. The difference is that I know you can do all of this *without dieting.* (Listen carefully and you can hear little angels singing.) So don't expect self-flagellation, self-denial, weigh-ins, wailing, and rabbit food for the forseeable future.

Instead, in 101 simple steps, I will show you how to:

* Stop judging and start living
* Eat more and weigh less
* Dress thin and look gorgeous
* Change your mind to change your shape
* Banish body blues and find body balance
* Realize that dieting is the problem, not the solution

This is a book with a realistic promise: It will examine your relationship with your fork, your fridge, your fashion, your friends, and your foibles. It nudges open the secrets of how you really feel about your body, and, in particular, those parts you'd rather lock in a box and never meet again. It looks at why we've become a nation of marshmallows, slumped in front of a computer or TV screen, and how we can ease ourselves off of the sofa and into a better body, while remaining—gloriously—within our comfort zones. And here's the icing on the cake: Unlike a diet, this book delivers effective solutions *today*—not tomorrow, not after the weekend, not when Christmas has turned into January. But now.

THE FAT OF THE LAND: HOW DIETING CONSUMED US ALL

It's odd, isn't it, that in a world beset by crime, poverty, hunger, an economic crisis, and a looming environmental meltdown, we should spend so very much time thinking about how much we weigh. It is, if you like, a metaphor for our times: While Rome, or its equivalent, burns, we're gazing at our navels and wondering who ate all the pies.

There are many curious aspects to our current obsession with body shape, but perhaps the most alarming is that the more we scrutinize the rail-thin celebrity A-list, the fatter we get. The gulf between the Eats and the Eat-Nots is now wider—literally—than ever. While a growing number of us are expanding at breakneck speed, the rest are panic-dieting, eating only grapefruit or protein or things that begin with the letter G.

For my part, I seem to have been on a diet since the moment my first child arrived—bringing with her a whole heap of joy, but leaving behind a whole lot of disheartening body issues: the heavier hips, the wider thighs, the belly hell-bent on heading south, boobs in close pursuit. Like many women, I have ricocheted between fashionable "It Diets." I've tried Atkins, Hay, Perricone, Caveman, Food Combining . . . I have done egg-white omelets, maple-syrup detox, cabbage soup in a Thermos flask, a Dulcolax at bedtime, an instant soup for lunch . . . Ring any bells? If there is one activity that really binds women together, it's our shared obsession with dieting. There is, after all, something hugely provocative about the possibility of losing weight, the promise that you'll actually shrink. It wins me over every time. And every time, I lose. Not weight, so much—mostly just the will to live.

DIETING?
THAT'S NO WAY TO LOSE WEIGHT

It doesn't take a genius to see the deep paradox at the heart of our modern relationship with food: The more obsessed we are with "healthy" eating, the fatter (and more miserable) we have become. For every "diet book" that hits the shelves, we put on an extra pound; for every "make me skinny" TV show, we let out our belts by one more liberating notch.

The average New Year's dieter cracks after 78 days—just, by some cruel twist, in time for Easter. All we know for sure is that dieting takes the fun out of eating. It leaves us lost. In fact, conventional diet strategies are believed to have a success rate of just 5 percent. There's such a wealth of evidence to support this cheerless fact that a team of psychologists at the University of California at Los Angeles (UCLA) conducted a comprehensive analysis of 31 long-term diet studies in order to unleash the inviolable truth. Their results, published in the April 2007 issue of *American Psychologist,* indicated that "dieting is actually a consistent predictor of future weight *gain*." The researchers wrote, "We asked what evidence is there that dieting works in the long term, and found that the evidence shows the opposite." The study found that, although people who go on diets can indeed shed several pounds in the first few months, the vast majority return to their original weight within

5 years, while at least one-third end up heavier than when they started the diet. All that willpower. All that punishment. All for nothing. The report concluded that it's better not to diet at all: "You're no worse off, and you spare your body all the damage associated with having a yo-yoing physique."

If you want fries with that, a 2003 study found that the more children and teenagers dieted, the more likely they were to become obese adults. Some experts now argue that obesity is increasingly a disease caused by its treatment. It is thought that parents who maintain and impose strict diets, or who engage in fad diets themselves, send the message to their children that food is dangerous, or something to fear.

In this climate of dread, it's hardly surprising that we're in a dieting-induced tailspin. For many of us, food is no longer a means of satiation and pleasure, but rather a source of guilt and reward. We wait, eager for the Next Big Idea (preferably with a celebrity fan-base) that promises to erase the love handle and the saddlebag, the muffin top and the triple-boob, or whatever new term the tabloids have thrust upon an innocent celebrity enjoying a day at the beach.

Your Body, Your Problem: How Food Became the Enemy

Part of the problem is that calories are everywhere, beckoning, beguiling. There are the happy hour specials, the buy-one-get-one-free sales. The Starbucks culture. The gargantuan portion sizes. We're short on time, so we drive rather than walk. We're short on expertise, so our evenings are punctuated by the ping of the microwave. We eat on the go or multitask during meals, picking up something we won't even taste, much less enjoy, and shoveling it in at traffic lights. (Consider the dispiriting thought that more Americans eat lunch in the car than in a restaurant.) Food is everywhere, and if it's not food profusion, it's food porn, turning our humble daily bread into something that now costs $10 at an artisan deli. No wonder we're overwhelmed.

And all of this, don't forget, comes in an era of food fascism, where every mouthful is graded and laced with guilt, an era in which women obsess about their bodies every 15 minutes (which is, apparently, more often than men think about sex). A third admit to using diet pills and laxatives, and 98 percent of us recently told a magazine survey that we *hate* our bodies.

The only comforting thing for me about all of this is that it's not just my problem. It's yours, too. We're all at it. The women I encounter in my travels as a fashion journalist often seem stricken by a paralyzing body crisis, spending their entire lives—the only lives they'll ever get, I might add—feeling bad because they're feeling fat. An unconscionable waste, sure; but you and I both know how real the body blues can be. I've been there. When I gained weight after having children, I felt dumpy, dreary, and about as sassy and engaging as a sofa. It seemed that my body shape could, with an extra pound here or there, dictate the very shape of my day. Like so many women, I spent years attempting to keep up, trying to slim down, poring over calorie charts, gleaning juicy little tips from celebrity trainers and Hollywood chefs, and using every ounce of willpower to stop myself from succumbing to the seductive powers of buttermilk pancakes or that last, provocative french fry.

But one day—a good day, a strong day—I'd had enough. I came to my senses. I'm still me, I thought. I'm just wearing slightly larger jeans. I looked at the research. Then I looked at my life, trapped between the bedroom mirror and the bathroom scale, eaten up with the dull minutiae of weight control. I realized that not only was serial dieting an appalling waste of time, energy, money, conversation, and emotion, it was also—ultimately—utterly pointless. That was the final ignominy of it all: In the long run, dieting doesn't work, won't work, can't work—and it will almost certainly leave us worse off. So I stopped. Right there.

At the same time, I started to write less about John Galliano's organdy kimonos and whether Prada made sense (the jury's out), and more about grittier, bread-and-butter issues: our connection with our bodies, our need to be a contender in the ring of perfect bodies, how our shape is changing (fast), why we're so very obsessed with dieting—and how, vitally, it just doesn't seem to work.

But if dieting was a fraud, then what *would* work? What could serve up the dream of slimness without the demands of Hay, Atkins, Zone, and the rest? What was needed, it seemed to me, was a live-it, not a diet: something practical, sustainable, effective, and holistic, even. What was needed was a way of life that viewed my appetite as part of a bigger picture, a realistic picture that encompassed my body image, self-esteem, lifestyle, and the regular ups and downs of my normal life.

As I began to compile this book, it became clear that the missing element in most best-selling diets is confidence. Self-esteem. Once you harness this magic ingredient—and this book will reveal how, in bite-size, transformative helpings—the slim you is a natural progression. In writing this book, I ditched the diets and started to find ways to feel better about being me. And guess what? I lost those last, pesky pounds.

THE 101 PROMISE

Here, then, is the no-diet diet. This book will help you lose weight—really—but it will also show you how to access your slender self. It is a book of directions, not rules. It's about tips and cheats, small things that collectively will make a big difference. There's a "mix and match" quality to it, partly because reading 80,000 words will lead you inexorably to the cookie jar—but mostly because some of the things detailed within will be your ticket out of here, and some just won't. Here are 101 suggestions to help you slim yourself down. It's a veritable smorgasbord of advice, and introducing even half of them into your everyday life (yes, your *everyday life*—this is no 2-week quick-fix, but rather a life-changing, never-going-back Thelma-and-Louise sort of book) will make all the difference in the world. Some are practical, others are psychological. Some are a bit of fun, some are a bit of work. There are new methods, and there is old wisdom. You'll discover a comprehensive examination of the artifice, the subterfuge, the tricks, and the illusions that are the staples of the fashion insider. These style and beauty tips will make you seem sensationally slimmer in an instant.

For every ploy, plot, and ruse to slim you down, there's a practical pointer that will make a tangible difference to your shape. There are countless simple strategies for calorie skimming, and an in-depth look at how your weight is ultimately, intimately related to how you feel. You'll learn how to normalize your relationship with food and why bringing it to the forefront of your daily routine, rather than tucking it in among all of your other responsibilities, might just obviate the need for serial-dieting, binge-eating, panic-snacking, and guilt-tripping. Oh, and it will also get you into smaller jeans.

This book encourages a commonsense, eminently feasible approach to weight loss. If you think it's time to free yourself from the billboard babes, from the tyranny of thin, from the curse of being on a constant diet, then this is the book for you. While we're at it, we'll also slaughter the diet myth, along with its inherent masochism and the self-inflicted misogyny it facilitates. This book will teach you to lay down your weapons and end the war with your own self-image. The first step is to start to love the skin you're in. Don't compare yourself to friends, sisters, celebrities, or that girl in your yoga class who always looks so great in lemon yellow sweatpants. It's a trap, and you could spend your entire life in that particular pit. Be kind to yourself, and you're on the first rung out of there.

In total, the 101 promise adds up to a rounded, comprehensive view of you and your weight, looking at ways to eat, ways to cheat, how to dress, what to ditch, and why you should thank your stars that you live in an age of Solution Lingerie. The journey will be positive, enjoyable, and progressive, and it will guide you to a place where you are happier, stronger, and freed from the shackles of thin and the torments of dieting.

In short, a "diet" isn't just about what you (don't) eat: It's about you, the whole you, and how you feel about yourself. Start understanding this, and you're on the way to figuring it out. Ready?

CHANGE YOUR MIND TO CHANGE YOUR SHAPE

❧ ❧

BODY BRILLIANCE STARTS IN YOUR HEAD

First things first: Do not stop eating! Isn't that a relief? But you *do* need to start loving—not that pretty cupcake, not those great ankle boots with the stacked heel, not J. Lo's new bangs, but *yourself.* Your head needs to be in the right place from the outset. So get it out of the sand (or out of the fridge—or, now that I think of it, out of that celebrity tabloid) and look in the mirror. This is where your journey begins; a little love and a lot of honesty will be your guides on the road to glory. This chapter is about reassessing your relationship with the world. It's about seeing sense, gaining perspective, and understanding what works for you. Not the girl in the lemon yellow sweatpants, but *you.*

1 DON'T READ DIET BOOKS*

It is a dispiriting fact that the greatest preoccupation of our age is with weight and its loss. As the world grows ever richer and rounder, we seem to grow ever more fascinated by the heft (or lack thereof) of our fellow men. Though, of course, we're far more interested in the women.

Think about how dieting and all its attendant nonsense have saturated our culture. How much time and effort it absorbs. We've trained ourselves to size people up in the blink of an eye. We're constantly aware of weight—its cruel lack or its licentious excess. We're hooked on A-list diets, quick-fix pills, self-help miracle cures, and the latest celebrity-endorsed regimes to issue from Los Angeles.

This, dear friends, is Diet Porn, a perverse phenomenon that undermines us all at a critical, visceral level. It gnaws away at our self-esteem as it sucks up vast tracts of time and energy that could be usefully expended elsewhere. While other eras basked in the Renaissance, the Golden Age, the Belle Epoque, we're lucky enough to have a TV schedule that boasts *America's Next Top Model*. Look, I'm not expecting us to spend our evenings ruminating upon the complexities of our being. But a little bit of thought beyond "Has she had a tummy tuck?" would make for a pleasant change.

The first thing you need to do, when building the platform upon which you will stand as you tackle the flabbiness that has crept into your life, is to Think Straight. You *have* to rid yourself of the dysfunction that marks our modern dance with diets. It's a ludicrous, exhausting gavotte, and it has to stop. You have to be in the right frame of mind. You have to sidestep the wild promises and wicked propaganda of an industry dedicated to keeping you in its grasp.

So stop staring at Gisele's butt and wondering how she does it, and start living. Stop measuring yourself against a warped societal norm, and start enjoying what you've got. Stop believing the barrage of misinformation

---

* *This, I hasten to add, is not a diet book. It is a "not-a-diet" book, designed to help you develop positive relationships—with your jeans, your butter dish, your waist, and your world.*

and what Susie Orbach calls "the fictions that dominate our culture." Start reading something edifying, instead. Get your sustenance from poetry, from Plato, from dancing the tango in platform heels, a red rose clenched between your teeth. Just don't get it from cake.

2 BELIEVE THAT YOU ARE BEAUTIFUL

You are already gorgeous. You just don't know it yet. To truly absorb this fundamental fact, you may well need to reset your Fat Goggles and recognize that carrying a few extra pounds is not a cardinal sin, no matter what the more pernicious quarters of the media would have you believe. Kerry Halliday, PhD, a London-based psychologist specializing in body-shape issues, says she regularly encounters women who are a perfectly normal, decent size, "and yet they've convinced themselves that a size 6 is fat! So many of the people I see are a healthy weight, but they have a fat head, full of fat thoughts. There's this constant dialogue of guilt. It's there when they go to sleep, it's there when they wake up, it's internal and introverted and isolating."

Enough already! Embark on the new-you project from a position of *strength*. Loving yourself doesn't make you a narcissist, it makes you a realist, armed and ready to resist the onslaught of our bizarre, thin-obsessed culture.

You do, however, need to be realistic about your expectations. I've known for years that I'll never be a size 4, let alone a size 0. I know that Kate Moss can do hot pants and I can't, that my thighs sometimes brush against one another like old friends, and that a miniskirt somehow makes me look maxi. There's something very liberating about recognizing these small facts, accepting them, and then—whoosh!—letting them go, like so many shiny helium balloons. You're suddenly free.

This doesn't mean letting *yourself* go, though. This project is not about giving in and giving up, installing yourself in the shadows and waiting for oversize sweaters to come back in vogue. No. This is a plan of action, a quest for change, a manifesto to celebrate all that is great about being a woman.

So accept yourself, right now. Don't live the dream, live the reality.

You're not Katie Holmes. You have a soft tummy. You wish you looked better in a bikini, but you accept that you don't. Watch those shiny balloons go, one by one. Pretty soon, you won't even know they were there. And remember all the while that the fat-cat dieting industry is founded upon the expectation of failure; you, my dear, should start with the bracing power of hope.

3 OPEN YOUR EYES AND RECOGNIZE YOUR WORTH

By and large—unless you have some karmic reason to believe otherwise—you only get one body. It may wax and wane, ebb and flow, but broadly speaking, you've been given those legs, that chest, those buttocks, this mortal coil—and you're not going to be issued another set upon request. Rather than poke your body in the eye with a fork, wouldn't it be better to love it, even just a little bit? But how can you love someone you don't really know?

Before you get started, you really need to understand exactly what shape you're in. Unless you turn on the lights right now, you'll never grasp the truth—so it's time to get a grip. Sneak a look; you won't bite. I'm not expecting you to conduct a microscopic investigation of every inch, but you do need to have a handle on how you really look, who you really are, and whether those wide-legged palazzo pants are really such a good idea.

So stop ignoring your reflection—in shop windows, in the mirror, in those brutal changing rooms where you catch a rare glimpse of your unfamiliar buttocks . . . because none of it is going anywhere unless you take notice. Look through vacation photos. Don't shy away from the truth—it's never as bad as you expect. (Though that bikini in Bermuda really *was* a shocker.)

Once you have had a proper gawk—yes, naked, with the lights on—you can start to weigh your options. I don't suggest you install vast mirrors on every available surface—the aim is not to make your home resemble a gentleman's club—but do administer a good dose of exceptional honesty. If you're the kind of person who likes to keep scrapbooks

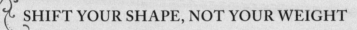

SHIFT YOUR SHAPE, NOT YOUR WEIGHT

It's worth noting early on that you—yes, *you*—don't really want to lose weight at all. What you want to do is *change shape*. If you are round and bottom-heavy, you want to be leaner. If you are wide and wobbly, you want to be taut and toned. I know, I understand—because I do, too.

The issue, then, isn't how much you weigh, per se. It's not even your BMI rating. This score (mine happens to be 21.9) is necessarily abstract, a general theory that cannot hope to measure the particulars and peculiarities of the individual. The equation used to calculate a person's BMI is:

Weight in pounds / (height in inches)$^2 \times 703$

Note that nothing in there accounts for body type, ethnicity, or composition—and as such this equation should be treated with informed caution. A perfectly fit, lean athlete can easily be classified as obese using this system. Need proof? According to his BMI, Brad Pitt is technically "overweight," while Arnold Schwarzenegger and George Clooney are both "clinically obese." Even Leila Ali clocks in as a heavyweight.

If you're seriously overweight, or just desperate to have a number stamped on your size, a BMI score may be of use to you. (Indeed, there is no real alternative that does the job any better.) But for a run-of-the-mill, slightly-on-the-chubby-side person, knowing your BMI is about as much use as knowing how to do quadratic equations. And when was the last time you had to solve one of those?

Far better to feel the real. Use your eyes. Use your pants. Use your unforgiving and not-entirely-kind mirror. We all know, for instance, that muscle weighs more than fat. We all know that fat located in certain areas is more troublesome to the eye than others. We all know that one woman's 150-pound hell is another's 150-pound paradise. Find your happy place.

and ticket stubs from amazing journeys, you might want to take "before" photos (it's probably best to keep these to yourself, though) so that you can marvel at the "after" shots in a couple of months' time.

Whatever you see, don't be mirror-miserable. If you face the music and feel fat, don't binge on shame and finger-pointing. You're only on Step 3. We've barely begun! Instead of seeking out and dwelling upon the downers, look for, and emphasize, your positive points, remembering all the while that you're never as fat as you feel. Your task—with the help of the next 98 steps—is to stop feeling fat and start feeling fabulous. Understand now (and recall often, as you read the next 10 chapters) that a gentle softness, a Rubens roundness, is feminine and beautiful and *absolutely* fine. It is infinitely more appealing than a desperate yearning for a flat stomach and toothpick thighs. (And if you find yourself doubting this for even a second, just ask a man.)

4 STOP WORSHIPPING *THIN* AND LOVE THE SKIN YOU'RE IN

It is hardly a revelation to note that as a society we are obsessed to the point of distraction by thinness—associating it, as a recent survey found, with "success." By the tender age of 6 years old, most girls are dissatisfied with their bodies and want to be thinner, according to research published in the *British Journal of Developmental Psychology;* almost half of those girls believe they need to go on a diet to lose weight. "Girls seemed particularly aware of teasing and likeability on the basis of weight and shape," the report concludes. [1]

The psychologist's explanation of this body-bashing is that, in these egalitarian times, when there are few remaining hierarchies based on religion, background, money, or education, we tend to judge people in terms of their appearance. Image is currency. Consider this fact: Until the seventies, only overweight women dieted. Today, only overweight women don't.

Of course, this book is all about putting an end to that. While there's nothing sinister or odd about wanting to feel fit and healthy and look great in a pair of shorts, there is certain danger in persuading yourself that all the troubles of your world could be eliminated if only you slimmed down. Life—fat, thin, or somewhere in between—will always have unpleasant surprises in store, whether you are 160 pounds or 115. Even at your fantasy weight, you'll still have to deal with your husband/teenagers/aggravating mother-in-law. There will still be bills and traffic jams and that annoying stain on the rug where you spilled red wine. You won't enter nirvana as you finally break into the 120s, so stop putting all of your hopes and dreams into one skinny little basket. Recognize that being thin is not the same as having a good body. Once you've gained perspective, you'll probably lose weight. Life's weird like that.

5 USE YOUR BRAIN, NOT YOUR FORK

Kooky as it sounds, you can "reprogram" your brain to eat well. Along with physiological demands, hormone surges, and social pressures, there is another influence at work on your appetite: Psychology.

A human mind is a lot like a human child. Tell it not to do something, deprive it of something (anything, really—*High School Musical* stickers, Spiderman lunch boxes, chocolate-covered macadamia nuts), and it will want that thing *more than any other little thing on the face of the earth*. It will obsess. Ever tried telling yourself "I must not have that cake"? Works about as well as telling yourself "I must not think of pink elephants," right?

In a study by psychologists at the University of Hertfordshire in the United Kingdom, dieting was actually found to *increase* cravings for "forbidden" foods, such as chocolate. In their experiment, researchers showed 85 women a series of images of enticing chocolate cakes and desserts drenched in fudge sauce—and they found that subjects showed significantly more desire for these than for other covetable objects displayed, such as perfume or a Mercedes-Benz. So far, so what? Well, among *dieting* women (those who had dieted in the last year or who were on a diet at the time), the responses were even stronger. They experienced heightened cravings and feelings of guilt. "Dieting appears to make a difference to how people perceive food, in this particular instance, chocolate," the study concluded. "Instead of helping people to

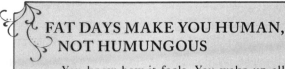

FAT DAYS MAKE YOU HUMAN, NOT HUMUNGOUS

You know how it feels. You wake up all wrong. Your face stares bleakly out from the mirror, demanding to know why you even bothered emerging from the sack. Your wardrobe is a freakish obstacle course, a land of booby traps and trip wires, filled with oddly shaped jackets and cheek-sapping colors. That dress you looked *amazing* in last Friday? Nightmare. The sexy, sultry siren shoes? Slutty. The red V-neck sweater, the one that made you feel like Marilyn Monroe? More like Marilyn *oh no*.

There are those days when the very same clothes you wore yesterday (on the very same body, of course) can feel inordinately different—and that difference depends entirely on something as insubstantial and subjective as your mood. We all have days like these. No one is immune to bad hair days, bad skin days, big butt days, days that seem to be full of snagged stockings, broken nails, and dashed dreams. They arise because we're human.

More to the point, they arise because we're women.

They're the unfortunate consequence of hormones, emotions, perception, a chance comment, an off look. These unfathomables can't be put on a slide and studied under a microscope. They can't be analyzed, dissected, and diagrammed. But intangible or not, they can have a potent effect on your day and how you feel about it. Accept them. Don't fight them. Today will become tomorrow, and that dress that makes you look like a pumpkin today may turn you into a princess then, just because you've *changed your mind*. Even Hamlet knew that "there is nothing either good or bad, but thinking makes it so." So don't read too much into your mood swings. Read Shakespeare, instead.

eat more healthily and to cut down on products which are bad for their health, the negative effect induced by dieting appears to have the opposite effect in that it can increase the desire for the actual foods they are trying to avoid. . . . If we constantly deprive the brain of the food we most desire we crave it even more." [2]

Clearly, you need to nip that right in the bud—first by allowing yourself just a little of what you fancy, and then by moderating your behavior around foods that will make you fat. As it turns out, "think thin" is not such an empty phrase. According to another recent report, it *is* possible to think yourself thinner. The study involved 47 women who were each asked to spend one half-hour thinking after having consumed a large lunch (something I've always found delightfully easy to do, though falling asleep is a constant threat). Researchers found that encouraging the subjects to remember the details of their last meal made them one-third less likely to eat snacks.[3]

Suzanne Higgs, PhD, of the University of Birmingham, who led the research, submits that this could point to a stronger connection between memory and body weight than previously thought. According to Dr. Higgs, "How well people can remember could be a factor in explaining why some eat more than others. There are certain things that we do now which are rather distracting and could stop people recalling quite as well what they have eaten."[4]

So pay attention. Watch what you eat, in a noninvasive, laid-back way—like a chilled-out parent keeping an unintrusive eye on their kid in a wading pool. Some people uncover the truth by writing a "food diary," believing that detailing their intake limits it and helps avoid "unconscious eating." You can try it; it doesn't work for me. (I did once write a food log covering the period between breakfast and lunch, and I found the experience so tedious that I turned to shortbread for solace and to add texture to my day.) But it may work for you. The idea, really, is to be conscious of what you eat and to know where your foibles lay, waiting to trip you up at the first tummy rumble.

Even if you don't buy the psychobabble, you can at least recognize that your ego, superego, and id need to be pulling in the same direction: toward a healthy, balanced, confident new you. You'll do much better if you stop punishing yourself about your body and the space it occupies. Punishment will only lead to rebellion and a recidivist streak, hurling you senselessly back toward the open fridge. Be kind. Think good thoughts. (But don't add fudge sauce.)

6 LAUGH AT CELEBRITY MAGAZINES

Open any weekly celebrity tabloid and you'll come across the usual parade of unnaturally thin women, their brows set in grim determination to avoid lunch. Over the past decade, many of our contemporary heroines seem to have reduced like stock on a stove until there's nothing left of them but skin and bones. It is this look, this *lack*, that has become an aspiration and inspiration for a whole generation of girls.

We've always admired icons, of course. Jennifer Aniston herself remembers idolizing actresses as a child. "Their hair, their clothes, their makeup were perfect," she told the *Observer.* "Looking back, I realize it wasn't a good thing. I was wanting to become this unattainable person." The consequence, she later confessed, was an eating disorder that wrecked her health. "I started taking vitamins and exercising and went too far. You get into that Zone Diet thing and you kind of get addicted to that." Similarly, Sarah Michelle Gellar has said that being a celebrity means inhabiting another space, another dimension—and that for a civilian to attempt to join in the charade is hopeless. "Look," she told *Vanity Fair.* "It's crazy for people to try to be as thin as we are. We have personal trainers and personal chefs. It's our job to look this way."

Clearly, there's no point even attempting to keep up with the weightless A-list—though many mere mortals, seeing the absence of proper female flesh up there on the pedestal of fame, will try. I've known this truth for years, of course—ever since, well over a decade ago, I stumbled upon the art director of *Vogue* magazine using a scalpel to carve a few centimeters off Claudia Schiffer's ankles. It was, I hasten to add, a transparency he was working on, not Schiffer herself, which would have made an awful mess of the parquet floor. But even so. I have always been pretty miffed that even Claudia—an original supermodel and all-around babe—wasn't deemed quite good enough for public consumption in her natural state.

In real life, of course, celebrities have to work their butts off (literally) to look even halfway gorgeous. If they ever stopped making an almighty effort, everything would fall apart, like a popsicle left out in the sun. I promise you, this is the truth. With all of the preening, pummeling, and primping that goes on, it's little wonder that most of them don't speak a second language, make their own jam, or play the piccolo. Keeping themselves thin simply takes up all of their time.

They do, however, have the time to follow zany diets based on spirulina (blue-green algae—sounds yummy, right?), bee pollen, and obscure Amazonian berries unavailable on the open market. It's all cayenne-pepper cordials and Myoplex protein shakes out there in the Hollywood Hills. Fridges are locked at night, and the key is sent home with the housekeeper. Trainers are on the doorstep at dawn, armed with grape seed extract and a 14-hour exercise schedule.

Sure, the bodies these women end up with are, very often, stupendous. But at what cost? Not long ago, an engaging picture turned up showing the chance meeting of Cameron Diaz and Victoria Beckham at the MTV Music Awards. Both had poured their golden-brown bodies into tiny little tubes that were, briefly, doing duty as dresses. At one end of the dress, the women were all naked necks and shoulder blades, taut faces, bronzed skin, and perky breasts. At the other end of operations, both wore painful-looking silver shoes, with heels and toes so pointy that that you had to wear safety goggles just to look at them. This, it struck me, is the modern uniform for celebrity dress-up. Perfect skin, muscular boobs, long limbs, wicked heels. And maintaining a body in such a streamlined state is clearly a full-time, staff-required, relentless job.

Such extreme maintenance has lately become the stock lifestyle in Hollywood and beyond, leaving folk like us languishing in the slow lane. Bombarded daily by these images of physical perfection, we've come to view these bionic women as normal. And so, while our glossy magazines

THE SIGH OF SIZE: HOW WE LOST OUR WAY

Twenty-five years ago, the average model weighed 8 percent less than the average American woman. (Yes, Twiggy was abnormally petite in her day.) Today's model weighs 23 percent less than the national average.

As long ago as 2000, the British Medical Association, in its report *Eating Disorders, Body Image, and the Media,* noted that the extreme thinness of celebrities was "both unachievable and biologically inappropriate," observing that the gap between the media ideal and reality appeared to be making eating disorders worse. "At present, certain sections of the media provide images of extremely thin or underweight women in contexts which suggest that these weights are healthy or desirable," it stated, recommending that normal women in the upper reaches of a healthy weight should be "more in evidence on television as role models for young women." Television producers and those in advertising should review their employment of very thin women, and the agency responsible for regulating what is broadcast on TV should review its advertising policy, the report recommended. Almost a decade on, and the opposite has happened.

Every now and again, someone inside the industry will take up the fight. Emma Thompson, for example, is known to be on a crusade against the idiocy of thin that plagues her profession—and she intervened when Kate Winslet (on the set of *Sense and Sensibility*) and Haley Atwell (on *Brideshead Revisited*) were encouraged by producers to shrink a couple of sizes. But this rebellion is the exception, not the rule.

Maybe it's time to step back and think about what has historically defined beauty. Back in 1913, *Webster's Revised Unabridged Dictionary* defined the word thus: "properties pleasing to the eye, the ear, the intellect, the aesthetic faculty, or the moral sense." Hmm. I'm not sure that a size 00 permanently hungry woman with a lock on her fridge door fits any of those criteria. Are you?

are populated almost entirely by waif-thin models and supernaturally tan celebrities, the back pages are dedicated to fat-busting fad diets, liposuction ads, and articles describing how meals that wouldn't satisfy a rabbit can turn you into a Glamazon in a single lunch hour (as long as you don't actually have any lunch).

In the process, many of us have lost all perspective, developing freakish ideas about what women are supposed to look like. Think of our screen stars, our pop-stars, any model on any catwalk anywhere in the world—I've got handbags that weigh more than they do. I could fold up someone like Eva Longoria and pop her into my pocket. In this Looking Glass world, a 90-pounder is a heavyweight. True perspective can be gained when you consider that the pinup of the 1890s was Lillian Russell—*all 200 pounds of her.* I don't even have to mention Jayne Mansfield, Rita Hayworth, Jane Russell, Sophia Loren, Raquel Welch—none of whom would get the job today—to prove that something's up.

To maintain this abnormal body shape, our icons—whether or not they're brave enough to step up to the plate and admit it—are permanently hungry. Elizabeth Hurley has admitted as much. Marcia Cross, who plays Bree Van de Kamp on *Desperate Housewives*, recently confessed that staying thin was "a living hell," and that she felt she had been banned from eating since joining the show. Actresses, models, singers, presenters—all are subject to the dictatorship of thinness enforced by the minders, molders, and producers who know very well what sells. It happened to Courtney Love and Carrie Fisher. I know from my experience in the fashion industry that it happens to hopeful young girls from the moment that first Polaroid is taken at the modeling agency. Christina Ricci recalls the favored put-down for wannabe actresses in Hollywood: "They say 'She looks too healthy,' which means 'She needs to lose weight.'"

It's a strong current, this grim undertow of the image game, and it's almost impossible to resist. Some try. When British model of the moment Daisy Lowe arrived in New York for her first season of shows, she was called "a little hefty." Her response? "I am who I am. My old agents in New York suggested I lose weight. So I moved agents. I'm extremely proud of the fact that I am two sizes bigger than most models. Being a stick is so unsexy."

Too true, though it's something that magazine editors are only slowly, gingerly, coming to realize. Says Sophia Neophitou-Apostolou, editor of *10* magazine: "The designers I work with now are demanding a more womanly girl (our struggle to find this is like searching for the proverbial

IT'S YOUR BODY, BUDDY: HOW TO NEUTRALIZE THE NEGATIVES

* **Heavy in the hips?** Well, so was Sophia Loren in her heyday. The trick here is to go for the cling, making a fuss of your bust and whittling away at the waist for that classic hourglass appeal.

* **Blocky in the shoulder?** Try a wrap, a plunge neck, or showing off some killer cleavage. It's how Jessica Alba and Helen Mirren get by, poor dears.

* **Short in the leg?** A boot-cut pant, a skirt that stops dead at the knee, a neat short-line jacket to lengthen a leg . . . all will help to stretch your proportions and add an illusory lift. It goes without saying that heels are your loyal ally. Eva Longoria in flats? I don't think so.

* **Piggy in the middle?** *Me too!* You don't need a tummy tuck, you need a tummy tamer, one of the many practical ways to scoot diplomatically over the issue. So drop your waistband or raise it to the empire line; choose tops with either a forgiving swing in the hem or the firm tailoring you want to keep you safely tucked in.

* **Broad in the beam?** Didn't keep Beyoncé and J. Lo off the map. Go an inch or two wider at the shoulder and the hem to make your waist work harder.

We'll expand on these issues—and dozens more—in Chapters 5 and 7, where you'll discover exactly how to dress to play up your personal positives.

needle in a haystack), and art directors are complaining that, these days, they're adding curves rather than shaving them off."

They do, however, want those curves in the regulation sexpot places, as Elizabeth Hurley recently discovered when her breasts were electronically enlarged for the cover of *Cosmopolitan* magazine. "On my last *Cosmo* cover," she told *Details*, "they added about 5 inches to my breasts. It's very funny. I have, like, massive knockers. Huge. Absolutely massive."

Right. So let's just admit that the inner sanctum of fame is a weird, airbrushed world. You, however, are not an inflatable doll, to be pumped up and down at will. Your challenge is to ignore these extremes and reacquaint yourself with the bell-curve of normal womanly weight. Real women are soft in places, and good to cuddle with. If the celebrity template starts to look reasonable to your eye, then stop looking. Shut the magazine. Go for a jog, instead.

7 FIND YOUR STRENGTH AND PLAY TO IT

While our forebears occupied themselves with the knotty issues of universal suffrage and how to feed a family of seven on a single turnip, we lucky, lazy 21st-century women spend a great deal of time pondering our own navels. A recent survey in *Grazia* magazine uncovered quite how spectacularly our bodies dominate our lives. Seven out of 10 of us apparently think life would improve greatly if we had a "good" body (world peace is so *passé*), and half of us think that our body shape and size spoils our sex life. (It's worth noting that most men would probably beg to differ; as Phil Hilton, former editor of the British men's magazine *Nuts*, once said on the subject of perfect boobs, "Men think all breasts are good and are delighted to have access to any at all. The idea that they are connoisseurs is inaccurate.")

Yet most women—and it matters little how educated, successful, or, indeed, beautiful we are—despair about arms that wobble, chins that double, and thighs that meet in the middle. Rather than look for strengths—our own and others'—we are continually on the lookout for weakness: the sweat-stain on the shirt, the spinach in the teeth, the cellulite peeking from beneath the miniskirt.

University of Leeds Professor of Medical Psychology Andrew Hill, PhD, believes that disliking particular body parts in this piecemeal, picky way is a modern phenomenon. "Now we have the technology to change specific areas of the body," he says. "We can be more hypercritical simply because we can fix the problem. It's all part of the new culture of self-improvement which wasn't around 30 years ago."

And so we chip away at ourselves, undermining our own confidence, sinking our own ship. The point is that we *all* have our unbecoming bits, the stuff we'd prefer to keep under wraps. Madonna, for instance, despises her chubby "Italian" thighs, inherited from her mother; George Michael's face is always pictured half in shadow because he doesn't much like the other half. And Kiefer Sutherland admits to keeping only one mirror in his house because he doesn't much care for his looks.

Drew Barrymore has mastered the art of strength-playing. "You learn to love your body," she says, with the wisdom of one who has been in the public eye long enough to get real. "You can't look at models and feel bad about yourself. I'm not the kind of girl who can stuff her face with pasta all the time and not gain weight."

Don't you just love that? Don't you want to give her a hug and buy her a hot chocolate (skinny, no cream)? Now then. On a personal note, seeing as we're all sharing, I'd like to introduce my not-quite-but-almost-perfect ankles. I got them genetically, along with a good ear, a decent singing voice, and a nose that gives generous shade on a hot day. So I wear fancy shoes, cropped pants, and lots of dresses, giving these ankles a lead role in my life. I'm comfortable in the knowledge that while they're dancing center stage, my less-excellent regions can fade unnoticed into the background.

My middle, for instance.

I am one of those women with a soft center. My stomach is squashy and yielding, like freshly baked bread, though resolutely stubborn in its refusal to budge despite the occasional desperate burst of sit-ups, curls, and the odd stern talking-to. It is my *bête noire* and cross to bear, this belly of mine. But have I mentioned my fabulous ankles?

See? Take a tip. You may loathe your shoulders, knees, or toes (though I'll put good money on it being belly, boobs, or bottom). But before you start prodding yourself with the vicious little stick of self-hatred, find the bit you love the most. Not the least. The *most*. If it's calves, show them. If it's cleavage, take the plunge. Don't point out your thunderous thighs and just hand ammunition to your adversaries; emphasize your pretty wrists, those full lips, that smile. Believe in your beauty, don't fixate on your foibles. And if you can make the most of what you've got with the judicious use of candlelight and high-waisted dresses, then so much the better.

8 DISCOVER YOUR OWN STYLE

What you wear is of absolute import and impact, your passport to a whole new world of thin. For every questionable bubble skirt, for every poncho in the "must-have color of the season," there's a piece of clothing that will make your body sing, simply because it nails your own unique presence, your sense of self. This, incidentally, may have very little to do with the trends of the day. Discovering clothes that work *with* you rather than fight against you is the fundamental principle of great style, and it's the linchpin of weight-loss dressing.

It's not just what you wear, but how you wear it that matters. It's in the tilt of your hat, the nonchalant throw of your scarf, the purpose in your stride. It's about risking a clash (it never did Yves Saint Laurent any harm) or perfecting a classic. (A tux for evening? A cashmere crew? There are very good reasons why these superior staples have been loved for so long.) Everything you put on gives off subtle signals, coded impressions that can captivate or caress a room—or turn it off like a switch. Your mission is to convey a message of confidence and ease. By the time you reach Step 101, I can guarantee that you'll have this self-possession, this poise, stashed in your pocket like a lucky charm.

For the moment, you need to know that, like much in modern life, it's all in the sell. Walk into that room like you own it, or at the very least like it owes you. Behavioral Analyst Sue Firth agrees that style is the consequence of confidence—available to anyone willing to make the effort, no matter what their age or shape. "It is about time-taking," she says, "about attention to detail. The whole impression sends out a message of charisma, and that is what we are drawn to. Projecting style is a function of confidence, self-esteem, and self-respect."

Rather than trying to find a new patent leather tote bag, try to find your *style*. Be true to you. As legendary raconteur and wit Quentin Crisp once said: "Fashion is what you adopt when you don't know who you are." So, if that trendy sweater makes your chest look like a sack of ferrets, ditch it. If the catwalk calls for white pants and your tush calls for mercy, give it a break. If you always get compliments in that subtle gray pantsuit, the one you've had for years, the one that adores you, like a faithful hound, then wear it, regardless of what the catwalk has to say about the matter. Don't be in thrall to fashion—instead, hum gently to yourself that just because it's in, it won't make you thin. As Ingrid Bergman wisely said, "Be yourself. The world worships the original." One of the best ways to do this is to embrace Step 9.

9 DEVELOP YOUR TRADEMARK LOOK— HATS, HAIR, CLEAVAGE, RED LIPS, YOU CHOOSE

A few months back, over coffee, my great friend Carla went through something of an existential *crise*, right here in my kitchen. "Who am I? Who *am* I?" she wailed, head in hands and one strand of hair (I couldn't help but notice) dangling perilously close to the cold coffee at her elbow.

"Ah, Carla," I said in my least patronizing tone, "As you get a tiny bit older, you can no longer experiment with every fashion trend, changing your haircut every third minute and expecting your body to settle into jeans or capris just because Marc Jacobs tells you to. No. What you need, as you age, is a Thing."

"A Thing?"

The congress of cold coffee and hair was now complete, and Carla was dabbing at the result with a Kleenex.

"Yep. A Thing. Like Debra Messing has all that fabulous red hair. And Jennifer Anniston's forever showing off those wildly perfect legs.

Nicole Kidman's got that ethereal white skin, and Anna Wintour has her blow-dry and . . . you need to find yourself to project yourself."

I was quite pleased with myself for coming up with this, but Carla seemed unimpressed. She sniffed loudly into the caffeinated tissue.

"But what's *my* Thing?"

"Go monochrome," I suggested brightly.

This is always my best advice to the lost sheep on the fashion farm. It's a tip I picked up years ago, when working alongside a particular fashion editor. Like all top-of-the-range stylists, this woman had access to almost anything her heart could desire. Trunks of Dior, towers of Versace, truckloads of Armani. Rhinestones, cashmere, wild silks from Samarkand, snakeskin handbags, Gucci shoes, Pucci pants. And what did she choose?

Black pants, white shirt. Every day. Religiously. She had obviously taken a vow, quite early on in her career, to "have a look"—a look, it has to be said, that owed more than a nod to the Albert Einstein school of dressing. (He kept seven identical suits in the closet and wore them in strict rotation, thus allowing his brain to settle on more taxing topics than whether his pants made his butt look big.)

This particular editor worked at the magazine every day in black pumps, exquisitely cut coal-black pants, and the kind of shirt that would glow in the dark, so clean and fresh was its whiteness. She always looked immaculate. (I actually suspect that she changed into an identical outfit after lunch, or whenever someone sneezed near her, or opened a purse.) There was none of that dizzy wheeling about in search of the next big trend; she did that for a living, so her own wardrobe simply maintained a calm decorum. It helped that she was gamine and adorable to look at, but her approach would pretty much suit anyone of a certain age who knows that her days as a hot, young thing are in the past.

Finding your Thing bestows upon you a sense of arrival, a feeling of strength and self-awareness. It feels like coming home. After much deliberation, Carla and I divined her Thing. Turns out she's a jingly jewelry sort of girl. She's going to wear charming bracelets that chime and clink as she walks, set against a sort of blank canvas of jeans, white T-shirts,

(continued on page 22)

WHO TO HIJACK: TOP CELEBRITY STYLE STAPLES

A trademark fashion staple is a little like having a personal assistant you can trust, or your own eyebrowist who understands the ins and outs of your face. They can draw attention to your fabulous bits or run interference for your dodgy bits. Think for a moment about the inhabitants of the world's "best-dressed" lists and you'll soon see that a signature is very often the element that separates them from the forgettable masses. The trick is to find—or steal—a style and stick to it, a bit like . . .

* **Elizabeth Hurley's white jeans.** She's worn them through thin and thin—even when they were about as fashionable as a paper bag. "I probably own 30 pairs," Hurley admits, "I love it and I know it works." Elizabeth is, of course, glossy and groomed enough to make white jeans look St. Tropez chic rather than shopping-mall trashy. But why does she wear them all the time? Because they have a strong style message: "I'm thin!" they cry, "And rich! I dry clean!" White jeans may not be quite your cup of tea—so experiment until you discover exactly what is.

* **Anna Wintour's classic bob and Chanel sunglasses.** If you are the most observed fashion plate on the planet—and, as editor of *Vogue*, how could you not be?—you need to manage the tightrope walk of style with consummate ease, and Ms. Wintour does, chiefly by relying on a signature triumvirate of big, bad shades, dead straight bob, and haute couture. I'm guessing your wardrobe is a little light on $40,000 couture pieces from Chanel—but a sleek haircut and a signature accessory? Those can be yours in a flash.

* **J. Lo's hipster flares.** Lopez, as we all know, has a glorious Latina butt, and hipster flares are a way of putting it up there in lights. We've all been fascinated with that rump for years; it's J. Lo's trademark. The flares maximize attention on those buttocks,

and—thanks to the additional material dancing about at ground level—exaggerate curves and generally look great.

* **Kate Moss's Very Important Pieces.** Consider what makes Kate's wardrobe tick: the Ossie Clark coats, the vintage rock 'n' roll jackets once worn by Keith Moon and bought at auction, the vintage thirties nightgowns, the "statement jewellery" that talks a hell of a lot more than she does. For all her style dipping, Kate is remarkably constant. She relies on quality, not quantity; buys originals, not knock-offs; and goes for authentic, timeless pieces, not poppy trends. She invariably attends business meetings in a Chanel power suit, "like Jackie O, but with a T-shirt, a power watch from Rolex, and my Vivienne Westwood Sex shoes." The point here is that she doesn't patrol the fashion landscape desperately picking up the latest bits of fluff to tumble off a catwalk. She knows her brand and she sticks with it.

* **Elle Macpherson's blazer.** An anachronism, perhaps, but being tall, Elle has the ideal figure for the coolly classic blazer. (Let's face it, she has the ideal figure for a Saks garment bag.) A blazer is, though, a forgiving staple for *any* shape—a snappy, practical wardrobe workhorse that can look particularly hot if it's worn a shade too small. (Shove up the sleeves for extra sass appeal.) If you're looking to copy Elle, avoid brass buttons and fire up your sober jacket with attitude; whatever mood you go for, avoid *smart*—you don't want to look like a prep school boy. The look you're going for is a bit AC/DC performing "Highway to Hell" in front of a stadium audience.

* **Audrey Hepburn's capri pants.** Cropped pants—to the shin or the knee—are a good way to show off delicate ankles and a pair of coquettish pumps. They're cute, too. Ever since capris first took off in the fifties, thanks to Audrey in *Sabrina* and *Funny Face*, the cropped trouser has suggested a carefree, run-along-the-beach sort of fashion freedom. If they could talk, they'd giggle and then smoke a cigarette (but not inhale).

and well-cut, expensive pantsuits. Genius, I think you'll agree.

No need to go mad, you see. Your signature could be something simple and chic (diamond studs, a slash of red lipstick) or something quirky and cool (high-top sneakers with your prom dress, a beehive with your ballet shoes, a bit of glitter and a lot of kohl). Personally, until I hit 38, I was all tawny hair and push-up bra. Lately, though, it's French navy, a becoming shade of teal, and an aquamarine ring that could double as an offensive weapon. For you, it may be a trench coat or perfectly tailored suits. It may be corsage and corsetry, or a crisp fitted shirt and bangles to the elbow. Whatever it is, find it. Wear it. Often. Not always—but often. Be remembered as the woman in white, the lady in red, the one most likely to succeed. Think of Diana Vreeland's rings, Katharine Hepburn's trousers, Coco Chanel's bouclé jackets, camellias, and pearls. If in doubt, find your icon—Monroe, Stefani, Jolie, Winfrey—and copy her. Style-jacking your heroine is no sin; it's the very axis of intelligent dressing. If Karl Lagerfeld can do it, then you can, too.

Don't, however, set your signature in stone and simply wait for death. Let it evolve, sticking to the general trajectory, but taking in the view along the way. Developing a Look, you'll soon find, is like developing armor; whatever the slings and arrows hurled at you, you're safe.

THE NO-DIET DOZEN

THE 12-STEP PROGRAM
TO FIX YOUR FATTENING HABITS

You've read all the books, you've clipped articles out of magazines, and you've tried to subsist on a handful of raisins and a couple of celery sticks. Well, me too. Having digested many a diet book on your behalf, I have identified the useful bits and put the rest out to compost. These are your golden rules, the 12 Steps that will whisk you from the dumpy ground-floor to the soaring penthouse in the time it takes you to read the chapter. With the following pointers, you'll have the basics for a new and healthy relationship with your fridge; by Step 21, you'll be well on your way to loving your own body. As Voltaire put it, "Nothing would be more tiresome than eating and drinking if God had not made them a pleasure as well as a necessity." So prepare to eat *more*, not less. (I told you this was a "no-diet" book.) Here's how to uphold the pleasure principle without busting a gut.

10 EAT A DECENT BREAKFAST

Skipping meals is never clever. Think about it for a minute, and you may be able to convince yourself that dropping breakfast will have you dropping a dress size. Tee hee, you'll think, no cornflakes this morning! That's saved me 150 calories and it's only 3 hours till lunch!

But think about it for 5 minutes and you'll soon realize that the opposite is true. The first thing you need to observe and understand is that you are an animal. Sorry, but you are. Deal with it. You have ancestors, sweetie. You, like me, started out in the primordial soup, and we're still carrying all the evolutionary baggage that got us out of there and into this incredible world of eyelash curlers and iPhones. This means that our bodies still respond to our environment in an age-old way, and no amount of wheedling or needling will change the way it does business. As countless studies have shown, skipping a meal—or going on any variation of the deprivation diet—merely evokes a primal "fear of hunger response," which will thwart any attempt you may make to lose weight. The basic biology of it all has been explained in full elsewhere, but, in case you've been living under a rock for years, I will give you a quick review of the basics.

* In times of food deprivation (for example, during the first desperate days of Atkins), the body's ancient hard-wiring kicks in.

* Your body—which really does have a mind of its own—decides it is being starved. Hmm, it thinks. No food. Where the devil will the next meal come from?

* Hormones rally. Worry not, they sing, we'll help you store some calories. We'll simply overrule the usual satiety signals, and we'll sharpen up those hunger pangs. Trust us, we'll get you through this!

* Anticipating further hardship, your body goes into squirrel mode, storing more food as fat and breaking down less of it for energy. It hangs on for dear life and, hungry as you may be, you'll *never* get to zip up that pencil skirt. This, let's face it, is not part of your game plan at all.

Unpredictable, unfulfilling, or omitted meals make you *hang on to fat stores* in anticipation of the next period of food scarcity (whether it arrives or not). Thus, most of the nonsense you find in diet plans will, by the laws of your very own body, backfire.

Further food for thought comes from a University of Nottingham study that found that keeping meal patterns constant also has definite metabolic advantages—associated with a greater "thermic" effect of food (the energy cost of its digestion and absorption), a lower caloric intake, and lower "bad" cholesterol.[1] For sustained weight loss, then, you need regular, reliable meals, best consumed in the following order.

A Good Breakfast

Breakfast kick-starts your metabolism, which has become sluggish and reluctant overnight, so it really ought to be treated like the most important meal of the day (and not just something you stuff in your face halfway between the shower and the train station). In a 5-year study of almost 7,000 men and women, researchers at Addenbrooke's Hospital in Cambridge, England, found that those who ate the biggest breakfasts put on the least weight over a set period, despite consuming more food overall each day than those who ate sparingly in the mornings. Cameron Diaz has taken this advice to heart and eats her dinner (garlicky lemon chicken with broccolini, since you ask) at breakfast time. Odd. But she says it keeps her going all day: "I started doing it when I'd go surfing because I could go out for 4 hours and not get hungry." Angelina Jolie did something similar to regain her killer shape after having twins. Her "upside-down eating" involved a vast morning meal (a full English breakfast, apparently), with calorie consumption petering out over the course of the day, ending with a small cup of homemade vegetable soup for dinner.

You, however, might prefer to go to work on a much more prosaic secret diet food: a humble bowl of oatmeal. This dynamite dish guarantees to keep you feeling fuller longer, particularly after exercise. Slow-burning, space-filling oats are formidable little power flakes, the food of Zeus. (They may even slow the aging process, which is information frankly too good to ignore.) While I'm all for oatmeal, it would help if you didn't add brown sugar, maple syrup, strawberry jam, or any combination of the three. Train yourself to like it plain. Jumbo oats make it more interesting; skim milk will, of course, slim it right down. Even better, make it with water, in the fine Scottish tradition. If you want to get really Scottish about it, you could always follow the Highland customs of the porridge pot: Some say it should only ever be stirred in a clockwise direction, using the right hand, so as not to stir up the devil; others contend that porridge should be spoken of as "they." And "they," by the way, should be eaten standing up. With a bone spoon.

If oatmeal doesn't do it for you, go for a decent slow-release, low-sugar muesli. If you have both the time and the inclination, make your own with oats, chopped nuts, an assortment of interesting seeds, and some grated apple. If not, you can have it custom-mixed in Austria to your exact specifications—adding Tibetan goji berries or taking out all the golden raisins; find out more at mymuesli.com.

The idea of all of this is to eat enough to preclude the need for a second breakfast at around eleven. You are not Winnie the Pooh. So, before you finish your oats and start loading the dishwasher, one more tip: Add protein. A recent study at Purdue University in Indiana found that eating a breakfast of eggs or bacon (or both) for breakfast elicited a greater sense of fullness throughout the day, compared to eating protein for lunch or dinner.[2] It's all in the timing. So add a slice of lean ham, a poached egg, a sliver of smoked salmon, green eggs and ham, a skewer of garlicky chicken—your choice—and it will set you right up for the day. Or at least until you eat . . .

A PROTEIN-RICH LUNCH

By rights, this should be your main meal of the day—so don't settle for a second-rate sandwich and a bag of chips. Go to town. Make a meal of it. Linger. I like the ayurvedic principle that we are designed to eat a larger meal in the middle of the day because our "digestive fire" is strongest between 10 a.m. and 2 p.m., allowing our systems to operate at peak efficiency. You may think this is nonsense. Fine—but do try to eat lunch at *lunch* time, won't you? Leave it any later, and studies show that you are more likely to consume a greater number of calories.[3] Do, however, bear in mind that glucose levels plummet post-lunch, so you might want to have a few nuts around for that mid-afternoon snack. (I recommend almonds, as you'll see in Chapter 4.)

A further word of advice: Institute a carb curfew after 5 p.m. With all due respect to dear departed Dr. Atkins, there *is* a time and a place for carbohydrates. Just don't eat too many, make sure they're the right, complex kinds, and eat them early. Why? Well, some dieticians say that the body will burn fat only after it has first depleted its store of carbohydrates, so why make night-carbs an obstacle to fat-burning? Others submit that our metabolism is in low gear at night and will tend to store late-day carbs as body fat. Some women report less bloating when they reduce their evening carb consumption. Whatever. The science isn't really firm on this one quite yet. All you really need to know is that if you cut back on carbs in the evening, you are likely to diminish your *overall* daily caloric intake without it being too much of a sacrifice. If, by contrast, you down a 12-inch pizza late at night, and then sleep on it? *Arrivederci*, skinny pants.

A SMALLISH SUPPER

The idea here, really, is to go easy in the evening; as the irritating old saying goes, "Eat breakfast like a king, lunch like a prince, and dinner like a pauper." The problem is that our culture, with its speedy days and lazier nights, its autopilot evening eating and its socially prescribed multicourse suppers, tends to "backload" calories at the end of the day. If dining out, we'll bravely embark on an epic journey from appetizer to coffee, taking in any sorbets, side dishes, and specials that come our way, as if doing so on a bet. At home, we associate evenings with wallowing in food and drink, and if we're not consuming, wouldn't we get a trifle, you know . . . *bored?* "Evenings are the time when most people munch on high-fat foods [such as cookies and other baked goods] because they are bored or tired," says Louise Sutton, a senior lecturer in health and exercise science at Leeds Metropolitan University in England. Okay. So, a carb curfew (see above) will head that off at the pass. (Eat a little more protein instead in the evening; it will help you stay fuller longer.) And if you're plagued by the soul-rotting ennui of an evening robbed of endless eating, just do something else—liberate your nights. Learn to tango. Play cribbage. Yodel. Embark on a journey through Dickens. Or just go to bed. Demote eating and start living.

One more thing: Eat supper at a reasonable time, leaving yourself at least a couple of hours to digest before you go to bed. That way, you'll sleep well and wake refreshed.

11 EAT *MORE* . . . OF THE RIGHT THINGS

Life shouldn't be an exercise in abstinence and deprivation. It should be fun and satisfying, and definitely full of food. What you need to know, though, is that everything works out fine just so long as you eat loads of some things and not a great deal of others. There's no mystifying formula to it, no secret recipe. We all know, deep down, what's good for us, even though the view may be momentarily obscured by a large slab of chocolate cake. Some foods are just more equal than others, and we have to nail the basics to have any hope of mastering the more challenging stuff to come. So, a few reminders.

* **Get complex.** Swap simple sugars for unrefined carbohydrates, which keep you going for longer, like the Energizer Bunny. Opt for carbs that are slow-burning (oats, basmati rice, whole-wheat bread) rather than fast-burning (brownies, muffins, anything made by Entenmann's). This is the best way to bypass the sugar cycle—the crave, consume, crash, crave, consume, crash spiral that we all know so well.

    The short explanation of how we end up in that spiral is that highly refined carbs, by spiking your blood-sugar levels, encourage your pancreas to produce insulin. Insulin, for our purposes, is your demon, your nemesis within. It's a cunning opponent, too, with more than one weapon at its disposal. First, it reduces the level of glucose in the bloodstream by diverting it into various body tissues for immediate use—or by storing it as fat. It also inhibits the conversion of body fat *back* into glucose for the body to burn. So insulin has a two-pronged attack: It facilitates the accumulation of fat and then it guards against its depletion. Insulin also acts on the brain to make you eat more, on your liver to manufacture more fat, and on the fat cells in your belly to store that fat. See? What a total fiend. A lovely, steady blood-sugar level—facilitated by those slow-burning carbs that take time and energy to digest—will stop your nervous system from demanding that you stock up on fuel. In other words, eat them and you won't feel as hungry. How simple is that?

* **Eat more brown food.** "People who eat white bread have no dreams," proclaimed Diana Vreeland. If you have ever attempted to create an interesting sandwich using a sliced loaf of white bread, you will see her point. The project is doomed from the get-go, even if you add tapenade or imported, cured meats. Even the term "white bread" has come to mean something bland and conventional, banal and tasteless. Why would you want to eat that? Brown bread, by contrast, is well-bred. If you haven't already made the switch, do so immediately. John Cusack, by the way, is said to avoid all white food—flour, sugar, rice, the whole lot. Most refined carbs are white, so it's a decent rule of thumb. If you can't commit to 100 percent brown, try bread made with naturally occurring white whole-wheat, which looks white and acts brown. (It doesn't have the tannins and phenolic acid found in the outer bran of red wheat, which some folks think give a bitter taste to whole-wheat products.)

* **Go for greens.** Yes, it's the old "fruits and vegetables" advice. But it bears repeating, because in addition to fiber and good vibes, fruits and veggies also contain vitamin C which, in addition to its many other health benefits, may well be crucial for weight management. According to researchers at Arizona State University, individuals who consume an adequate amount of vitamin C burn 30 percent more fat during moderate exercise than those who don't get enough of the stuff. They also showed that too little vitamin C in the bloodstream correlates with increased body fat and waist measurements.[4]

So go to it, remembering that vitamin C is fragile and easily lost. That means that if you're cooking your vegetables, do so quickly and tenderly.

✳ **Pick purple.** If you want to be truly in step with fashion (and Mariah Carey), go mauve. It will instantly increase your vitamin intake. Beets, eggplant, blueberries, açai berries, plums, purple carrots, purple cauliflower, figs, olives, purple asparagus . . . purple foods are thought to be naturally among the best sources of antioxidants and vital vitamins, and they should be added to your menu along with greens. As Mariah herself says, "I used to wake up and say, 'What do I want to eat?' Now, rather than order any old thing that tastes good, I'll say, 'What will keep me at the size where I feel better about myself?'" Borscht, that's what!

✳ **Learn to love the lentil.** Sadly, lentils have had a bad reputation ever since the hippies of the sixties appropriated them and based an entire philosophy on their simple, peaceful appeal. Lentils, together with other beans, have been part of the human diet since Neolithic times, and with good reason. In the Bible, Esau was tricked into selling his birthright for a pottage of lentils (Genesis 25:34)—and really, who could blame him? They are packed with protein, fiber, vitamin B, and other absolutely vital stuff such as iron and folic acid. Little legumes like lentils, chick-peas, and other varieties of dried beans, though unassuming on the shelf, are dynamite in the diet—in soups, in veggie burgers, in any number of glorious Indian dishes—deftly balancing blood-sugar levels while providing that all-important steady, slow-burning energy. What's more, there are so many to try: brown ones, red ones, yellow ones, and green ones. There are golden ones and black Beluga ones, and even a big yellow Mexican one called Macachiados. My favorite, though, is the funky little Puy lentil, which does all the stuff your average lentil can do, but manages to be fashionable at the same time.

✳ **Widen your repertoire to include grains you've not yet encountered.** Instead of relying on wheat—such a cliché—be wild and promiscuous in your grain consumption. Go for the wholesome whole ones, which boast way more micronutrients and fiber than their stripped-down cousins. As you search for interesting slow-release energy foods, try spelt, quinoa, bulgar, and buckwheat. Too humdrum? Flirt with amaranth or teff. You'll find these in health-food stores, and you can chuck them into salads, soups, and stews, or serve them as jaunty side dishes to impress your friends. Or, if that all seems like too much to contemplate, simply swap your refined white rice for brown rice. There are so many reasons to do so, not the least of which is this: Brown rice *actually tastes like something.*

12 EAT MEALS, NOT SNACKS

A moment, now, for memories: Do you remember packed lunches? My mom, like yours, made them at home, spreading peanut butter and jelly on bread and wrapping it in aluminum foil so it didn't leak in transit. Long ago, sandwiches weren't anonymous and ready-made, housed in a pyramid of plastic and containing all manner of fancy stuff, such as pine nuts. They were personal enough to allow you to compare fillings with your neighbor at lunchtime and swap peanut butter for tuna salad, if you both agreed. This, you may remember, was a time before salsa and pesto, before focaccia, caramelized onion relish, and hummus. Personally, and I am going back a bit here, I vaguely remember an era when salad was called lettuce, not greens; when balsamic hadn't yet oozed like edible crude oil all over the national palate; when we took hard-boiled eggs and saltines on long car trips in case we got hungry on the way.

I suspect that no one hard-boils eggs as frequently as they used to; we simply don't need the convenience they offer, since we get it elsewhere—from a compartmentalized plastic tray of Lunchables, perhaps, or a packet of string cheese. In my view, this is a great shame, as an egg is a perfect thing, a peerless marriage of protein and design. You simply cannot say the same of a shrink-wrapped stick of beef jerky.

While we've been distracted, working our way through the wondrous new and ever-widening smorgasbord of food on offer, what we eat has changed beyond recognition. While much of it gives good reason to rejoice (California rolls! Arugula! Eleven different types of olives!), the evolution of our eating habits has meant we eat more. More food. More snacks. More of the time.

Not only are our servings bigger, with everything available "deep dish," "super size," or "grande," but also, between bucketfuls, our propensity for snacking is extraordinary. Today, there are very few stretches of time that remain food-free. A business meeting? Hey, have a muffin. Waiting for a bus? Grab a cookie. Stopping for gas? Don't forget the donut! Run your eye along the snack aisle of your local supermarket and you'll be amazed by the breadth of choice out there. "King Size" candy bars. Crab-flavored potato chips. Teriyaky-style beef jerky.

For a little perspective, consider the fact that Americans spent more than $21 billion on snacks in 2006, consuming around one-third of all snacks produced in the entire world. That's a lot of grazing. This snack fest has changed the very shape of our days, with sociologists reporting that Americans have added to the traditional big three "eating occasions"—breakfast, lunch, and dinner—an as-yet untitled fourth that lasts *all day long*. One study from Harvard found that Americans are not consuming any more calories at mealtimes than they did two decades ago, but they have almost doubled their consumption of calories from snacks and carbonated drinks between meals.[5]

These devilish bites are what the food industry calls "ambient foods," designed for "transient" consumers who crave instant gratification. Trendwatching.com, a company that monitors and labels these things, calls this our Snack Culture, noting, for example, that U.S. sales of 100-calorie packs of crackers, chips, cookies, and candy grew nearly 30 percent in 2007.[6] At this point, it's worth noting the recent Dutch study that found that fun-size snack packs in fact encourage you to eat *more*, not less; participants who ate from "guilt-free" mini packs ate more because they were not exercising the self control demanded by a bigger bag.[7]

Here's even more food for thought.

* **The following things are not food, so don't put them in your mouth:** "handheld snacks," "portable snacks," and "snack kits." If you can pick it, dip it, pop it—do yourself a favor—drop it. Similarly, if you have to unpeel three layers of advertising to get at the food, it's probably not worth the bother.

* **Try to eat at a table.** And no, as Michael Pollan rightly points out in his brilliant book *In Defense of Food*, your desk does not count. Today, for many, the concept of a "family meal"—served at a table, with proper knives, forks, and conversation—is as old-fashioned as the concept of darning socks or making a bed with hospital corners. We have become a microwave- and freezer-based life-form. Introducing a table into the proceedings not only upgrades the whole experience, it also makes you mind your food. This is good. Remember that only animals eat standing up. If you're forced, by dint of deadlines and the demands of your day, to eat lunch at your desk, surprise yourself with a change of plan. Instead of trooping up to the closest sandwich franchise for one of those fat, mayonnaise-laden numbers, go one more block to that Italian deli or Spanish grocery on the corner. Buy a few slivers of exotic ham, a handful of salty black olives, a vine of plum tomatoes, and some bread for dipping into delicate green virgin olive oil. Let your screen saver gaze on in envy as you enjoy a proper little feast. Yes, it took longer to assemble and longer to eat, but you'll still remember it come quitting time.

* **Try not to eat alone.** Left to my own devices and free from the scrutinizing glare of my husband, I have been known to eat an entire family-sized pizza, starting at 12 o'clock and working my way clockwise all the way around to noon again. Alone, a human is like a hamster and will happily travel from one end of a tube of Pringles to the other without pausing to blink. Eating with company, by contrast, helps us restrain speed, slovenliness, and wanton behavior. (As one who has tried it, I can vouch for the fact that it is embarrassing to have thirds in front of guests.) Do bear in mind, though, that if you sit down with gluttons, you will almost certainly turn into one, too. If you have a large friend, invite her to the gym for a yoga class, not to your home for a pizza.

* **Avoid enormous food.** I am constantly vexed by the buckets of popcorn we're forced into buying at the movies. No one needs that much popcorn. Not ever. Not even to get through a Tom Cruise film. Broadly speaking, if the container is bigger than your head, don't buy it. (You'll save yourself at least five bucks in the process.) I am fond of the experiment performed by Brian Wansink, PhD, and his team at Cornell University; it involved giving Chicago moviegoers tubs of 5-day-old popcorn. Some got it in medium-size buckets, others in large buckets. The leftovers were weighed at the end of the show—revealing that the people with the bigger buckets of stale popcorn ate 53 percent more than the ones with smaller tubs.[8] They did it *because it was there*, which is pretty much why Mallory climbed Everest, but without the cardiovascular benefits. As the *New York Times* explains, "People didn't eat the popcorn because they liked it. They were driven by hidden persuaders: the distraction of the movie, the sound of other people eating popcorn, and the Pavlovian popcorn trigger that is activated when we step into a movie theater. . . . "

* **Leave plenty of time.** If you're in a rush, you'll never make yourself a healthy sandwich or an interesting three-bean salad. You'll stop off at the gas station and buy a Kit Kat. You'll also be bound to "inoculatte," which, according to the *Washington Post*, means "to take coffee intravenously when you are running late." Don't.

* **Plan ahead, and you'll cut back on snack attacks.** What will you eat tomorrow? What's for lunch? Is there any of that guacamole left? Tune in to your fridge and your kitchen cupboards so that you can make informed decisions about your meals. Don't just bump into food by accident, grazing on empty, worthless snacks. Don't allow yourself to be ambushed by dinnertime; it happens every day, give or take, so be prepared and make meals you love to eat. If you don't, that chicken chow mein take-out, that package of chocolate chip cookies, that bag

of chips will suck you in and spit you out on the wrong side of your new jeans, guaranteed.

13 OMIT NOTHING, FORBID NOTHING

Life is not an endurance test, so don't set yourself ridiculous targets. You will fail. Take your time and you will win, Grasshopper.

Try a bit of self-help psychology when you're struggling with the temptation of that beckoning donut. Tell yourself you can have it, but you don't really need it. Not now, at any rate. You can have it later, if you still want it. By that point the craving may well have passed. Or you will have moved away from the bakery window and gotten on with your life.

If you simply can't resist, if the glinting sugar and the chewy dough

DETOX, SCHMEETOX

You already know that you don't need to diet. What's more, if you eat a healthy, comprehensive, and varied array of nutrients, you do not need to detox, either. One of my favorite quotes on this topic comes from Andrew Wadge, PhD, chief scientist at the U.K. Food Standards Agency. He has urged people to ditch detox diets and supplements, writing on his FSA Web site blog that, "There's a lot of nonsense talked about 'detoxing' and most people seem to forget that we are born with a built-in detox mechanism. It's called the liver. My advice would be to ditch the detox diets and supplements and buy yourself something nice with the money you've saved. Personally, I would recommend the new Neil Young and Steve Earle albums."[9] What you need (and a Neil Young album might well help), is to ditch dysfunction and discover a healthy balance that works for you.

prove too much to bear, grant yourself amnesty. But don't use an accidental run-in with a bag of chips as a reason to binge until further notice, weeping as you shovel ice cream into your mouth. It was a blip, not a felony. Rather than admonish yourself, rather than prohibit, you need to forgive, forget, move on. To Step 14, perhaps.

14. COOK MORE. MAKE FOOD YOUR FRIEND, AND IT WILL LOVE YOU RIGHT BACK

Let me introduce you to Marcie, a dear friend of mine. Marcie sleeps between Calvin Klein sheets, has exotic flora in crystal vases dotted around her apartment (which happens to be in London's Primrose Hill), enjoys regular facials with someone called Aurora, boasts her own Pilates teacher, wears ridiculously expensive cashmere, and uses a pricey moisturizing gel on her sensitive eye area. Her kitchen is impeccable, full of professional-grade versions of all your standard appliances, not to mention an espresso machine, teppanyaki grill, and brushed-aluminum wine cooler. Her empty dishwasher (always empty) smells of lemons. Her white bone china is stacked in pleasing towers, waiting to be called upon for duty. Marcie's impressive pull-out cupboards show off their contents to the laziest eye—whole nutmegs, aromatic cloves, a weird herb called Nigella (bought as a token of her affection for England's greatest cook). But get this: She never uses *any of it*. Not the cumin, nor the coriander seed. Not the dried dill, the oregano, the saffron stalks that look like golden eyelashes. Marcie, though her kitchen screams gastronome, doesn't cook. She orders in; she eats out. But she doesn't cook. It reminds me of Jennifer Aniston's wonderful comment when she had just moved into her marital Malibu mansion with Brad all those years ago: "Staying in is the new going out. It's nice to invite your friends over, have dinner parties, play poker. Not that I can cook, but I'm planning on learning and we have a great kitchen."

We may not be as detached from the front lines of cooking as Jen or Marcie, but many of us have developed a perverse relationship with our plates of late. According to a recent study conducted by researchers at the University of Arizona in Tucson, Americans may love their food, but they throw out $43 billion worth of it each year. That's about 14 percent of what is bought.[10] And while we devour TV cooking shows, we have forgotten how to cook. Even if we're confident in the kitchen, able to pirouette between the béchamel sauce and the brûlée torch with the assurance of a pro, who isn't too tired, too busy, too idle to pick up a potato peeler at the end of the day?

Well, if we want to lose weight, to eat well, perhaps we should actually make an effort. There is, after all, something so vital, so visceral, about cooking. I don't expect you to skin a rabbit or hang a pheasant. And as a working mother I recognize how very easy it is to let it slide—how tempting a frozen meal can seem at the end of a hectic day. But stripped of its jazzy sleeve, what have you got? A beige lasagne made in a factory? Some anonymous mush ladled from a steel vat by a guy in a hairnet? Come on. Faced with the prospect of a microwavable meal, it's important to think outside the box. Perhaps not always, but often. How hard is it for me to put a chicken in the oven, a squeeze of lemon and a rub of sea salt on its chest? Could I wash some lettuce? Make a dressing with Dijon mustard, olive oil, and sharp white wine vinegar? Compared with ready-made meals, is there really a contest?

To really get a handle on your love handles, then, you need to come to grips with your food. Your dinner shouldn't say *ping!* It should say *mmm.* So follow Kelly Osbourne's advice and chuck out the microwave (ensuring no one is standing beneath your window first). Make a vow to develop a more intimate relationship with your food. Reconnect. "Food!" we should think at the appropriate hour of the day. "Delicious!"

15 GO SLOWLY AND DIGEST YOUR FOOD PROPERLY

It seems a simple enough invocation, but just think about how much you bolt. Gulp. Rush. British media personality Janet Street Porter's

FAST FOOD: HOW TO TELL IF YOU'RE SPEED FEEDING

✳ If you are talking with your mouth full, you're going too fast.

✳ If you get hiccups, you're going too fast.

✳ If you ask for the bill before you've finished your cheesecake, you're going too fast.

✳ Ditto if you spill things down your front, can't remember what you had for lunch, take a phone call during supper, or if your lunch hour lasts 12 minutes.

✳ Finally, if Pepto-Bismol is a staple on your grocery list, you are going too fast.

All of these things are signposts that you are eating too quickly and that you are unlikely to digest your meals efficiently. This is not only a problem for anyone who has to dine with you, it is also a big issue for your poor afflicted innards, and it can have a deleterious effect on your weight.

advice for a long and healthy life really ought to be emblazoned on your forehead in felt-tip pen: "Eat as slowly as you can and never miss a meal." This advice is increasingly important in a culture where everyone is always, always late. Just as Slow Food—the international movement opposing fast food and promoting dining as a source of pleasure—has taken hold in the collective consciousness, so Slow Eating ought now to settle in for the duration. By this I mean eating with intent. Eating to savor. History students among us will doubtlessly recall that witty aphorism, "nature will castigate those who don't masticate," the catchphrase of early diet guru Horace Fletcher, a fastidious fellow who promoted the idea that properly chewed food lessens the appetite, leading to weight loss and better health. Fletcher advocated chewing 32 times—or until the food became liquid in the mouth—before swallowing. He even suggested that *liquids* be chewed to mix them properly with saliva. Henry James and John D. Rockefeller were both advocates, and probably made for quite dull dining companions as a result. But Fletcher *was* on to something: Your mouth has a job to do in the breakdown of incoming morsels. Rush food through as if it's on a bullet train to nowhere, and you are asking for trouble. So do chew a bit more. And don't gobble, guzzle, wolf, or swig. Make a conscious effort to taste and savor your food. Put your knife and fork down between bites. Let your body know what's just hit it. Proper chewing is said to be the cheapest form of weight management, and if that doesn't sell it to you, nothing will.

While we're on the inside looking out, do try to get regular. I lived through the seventies, when every third person was on a high-fiber diet, eating tons of bran buds in a bid to convey food from one end to the other without impediment. There's still much to recommend fiber: It is found in the cell walls of plants—in fruit, vegetables, whole grains, cereals, nuts, seeds, and beans—and is not digested when we eat. This means it is an ideal bulking agent, making us feel full sooner and staying in our stomachs longer than other foodstuffs. It slows down our digestion rate—more lovely slow stuff—which means we stay full all the way from one roughage encounter to the next. (It is well known, for instance, that whole grain bread is twice as filling as the bland white alternative.) And, as an added bonus, fiber escorts fat through our digestive system, meaning that less of it is absorbed and lodged in the body. It is also a widely accepted (though little discussed) fact that at any given moment a quarter of the population is suffering from constipation. Nix it by hydrating, walking, and eating bran. Going slow is all very well in the kitchen, but not in the bathroom.

16 GIVE FOOD YOUR UNDIVIDED ATTENTION

Don't read, watch TV, text, drive, or juggle as you eat. That way, you'll know when you're full (at which point . . . *stop*).

HOW NOT TO EAT: YOU KNOW YOU'RE NOT ENGAGING WHEN . . .

* You find crumbs in your keyboard.

* The novel you're reading boasts thumbprints of jam on page 32.

* You have mastered eating while applying lipstick or (God forbid and forgive you) in the bathroom.

* The person on the other end of the phone says "Are they sour cream and onion?"

* There's a Ben & Jerry's Chunky Monkey stain on your nightie. (This is called "negligence" in our house.)

* The Sudoko is finished by dessert.

* You use three implements during supper: knife, fork, and remote control.

* Your partner says "Do you want any more pasta?" and you say "What pasta?"

* You shift your gum to one side of your mouth so you can eat a croissant.

In Japan, it is apparently considered rude to eat and walk at the same time, but somehow in the West our paths are populated by pedestrians stuffing in a muffin en route to somewhere vital. I am constantly amazed by the number of people who manage to eat on the run. Noodles with chopsticks. Whoppers with extra cheese. Pizza, ribs, burritos. All leaking onto the shared space of the bus seat or unsuspecting fellow passengers everywhere.

If you want to develop a healthy, skinny relationship with your calories, give them a little space. "Eating and drinking aren't errands," says the author of *The Fat Fallacy*. "It's not what you do on the way to something else." [11] Correct. It's something you do when you're hungry (not fidgety, not sad, not celebrating a great day, but *hungry*). Too many of us eat on autopilot, in a daze. One in five of us snacks when we're bored; most of us will eat until a TV program ends; some of us don't even know what's on the fork.

17 PLAY STRAIGHT—ELIMINATE ILLICIT FOOD STASHES

I'm talking about the Hershey's bar in the fridge, the cookies stashed in the bottom desk drawer, the gummi bears in the glove compartment. De-cache. De-stash. Pretzels under the bed? Bite-size Snickers in your pocket? Stop hoarding food for future use. If you're the kind of person who ferrets food away, keep it on a shelf, instead, like an ornament, not hidden behind a cushion on the sofa. Fashion designer Karl Lagerfeld, a man whom I adore despite his fantastic oddness, is said to keep "red meat, alcohol, and chocolate at home as a decorative accent to smell and see, but not eat." Note: Do *not* do this yourself unless you are already fantastically odd. Do, however, come clean. Be up-front, out, and proud, and rid yourself of guilty secrets.

Be aware (not obsessed, just aware) of what you eat on a daily, drudging, "whoa-did-I-really-eat-that-last-donut?" basis. In surveys, half of us admit to lying about how much we eat and to eating in secret. All over the country there are women, lodged in the pantry or behind a conveniently large potted plant, cramming in the last of the fudge while backs are turned. I do it. You do it. One poll found that 50 percent of women confess to having eaten an entire package of cookies in one sitting. There is, then, a below-the-radar food-fest going on in the kitchens, pantries, and utility rooms of the land. If you're at it, be aware of it.

18 SURPRISE YOURSELF; BREAK THE HABITS OF A LIFETIME

Studies reveal that up to 45 percent of what we do every day is habitual— performed without thinking, in the same location, at the same time, in the same dullard way. Think about the urge to check your e-mail. To wipe a counter. To apply lotion. To grab a cookie. It's why advertising works. It's why you trek through the supermarket each week on the same established route. "Habits are formed when the memory associates specific actions with specific places or moods," says Wendy Wood, PhD, of Duke University in North Carolina. "If you regularly eat chips while sitting on the couch, after a while, seeing the couch will automatically prompt you to reach for the Doritos." Now that we've hit Step 18, it's high time to change the schedule. Get random, have chance encounters, leave room to maneuver and space for the unexpected. Fight the triggers of habit, and you'll fight the fat.

"On a neurological level," says psychologist Kerry Halliday, PhD, "women plagued by weight issues need to develop positive pathways, not retread the negatives. It takes 21 days to break a habit—so, at first, every time you face a compulsion to eat too much, or to eat poorly, you need to face this head-on. Try to install a behavior that chips into your established route. Go for a walk. Phone a friend. Get out of the house. Leave your desk. Divert attention, break thought patterns, and change the picture."

We all, however, possess a "status quo bias," our everyday lives set to a well-thumbed default position. We head for the same seat on the bus, we stay with the same TV channel as one program segues into the next, we sheepishly follow the path of least resistance. What you need, then, is a series of minor movements. Small changes. No obsessions, but real differences. Stir it up, little darling, stir it up.

* Park as far away from the supermarket/work/bakery as possible. That way—guess what?—you have to walk farther.

* If you habitually eat in front of the TV or your computer screen, outlaw both. Be radical. Commit yourself to never again eating in the office, at your desk, or on the sofa. In a week or so, your habit—that regular, routine food-fest that you barely notice—will be reformed. Plus, you won't find cracker crumbs in your keyboard or lodged down the back of the sofa.

* Plot your pitfalls. Note when your self-control is likely to crumble. If you're always starving when you get home from work, make sure

there's a banana stashed in your bag to eat on the bus. That way, you won't demolish a whole loaf of bread as soon as you're through the front door. If you're prone to a late-night forage in the fridge, run a bath, instead. Avoid the traps—the foolish peering into the fridge looking for inspiration, the cupboard shelf stacked with chocolaty goodness, the evening wine bottle stationed so conveniently on the coffee table. If the kitchen is on your left, turn right. You may find yourself staring at a bookshelf, instead, or on the patio talking to a neighbor about cherry blossoms.

* Don't plant yourself in a forest of calories and hope for the best, for verily you will grow fat and complacent. Adjust your life to dodge your food fetishes. If you can't go into Starbucks without buying a blueberry scone (460 calories), don't go into Starbucks. If you pick up a candy bar every time you buy a newspaper, have your newspaper delivered. Study the enemy and don't put yourself in the line of fire.

* Consider your own personal Habit Map—the locations that, without fail, strand you in a whole heap of superfluous food. My own map would go something like this (giving both the enemy's coordinates and weapon of choice):

> **Dunkin' Donuts:** chocolate glazed cake donut
>
> **Starbucks:** Rise & Shine muffin and decaf tall cappuccino with extra foam
>
> **McDonald's:** chocolate shake
>
> **Panera:** cinnamon crunch bagel with cream cheese

And so on, my entire day punctuated with excuses to stop off and revisit an old favorite. Your mission, should you choose to accept it, is to break these habits. Take another route to work. Walk on by. Shop elsewhere. Cross the road when you know there's a food grenade in your path—an all-day breakfast, say, or an espresso stand that does a quite brilliant *pain au chocolat*.

* Get a handle, too, on your Food Memory Map—the behavior around eating that stems from your background, your childhood, the Proustian moments you may have stored in the dusty back rooms of your mind. It

may not be madeleines. It may be KFC or an entire tray of brownies. It may be potpie or lasagne or the petit fours your grandmother served on doilies in the dappled light of her front room. These sentimental delights are sewn into your soul, right in your cerebellum, the deep-buried primitive part of your brain, and your reaction to them now, as a grown-up, is a potent one. It's enough to have you reaching for an extra dumpling simply because it makes you feel safe and loved and liberated from the constraints and concerns of adulthood. Just be aware, that's all.

19 TACKLE TEMPTATION HEAD-ON

Ah, we all know how easy it is to make soaring promises about how little we'll eat tomorrow, how far we'll run next week. A Marathon in March! Rice cakes all weekend! It is considerably more difficult to modify your present-tense behavior—to get off that couch, right now, before the commercial finishes—than to plot your future brilliance. This is what social psychologists call "dynamic inconsistency"—the gap between what you plan in good faith and what you do in real life. The issue, as Richard H. Thaler and Cass R. Sunstein demonstrated so deftly in their hit book *Nudge*, is that humans respond to a given situation based on their state of arousal, whether they are "hot" or "cold." When in the cool, disinterested state, we tend to underestimate the effect of arousal. It's all very well to hatch plans to lose 15 pounds with the Just Say No principle, but when confronted with a bowl of french fries—tempting, crisp, and salty, right from the fryer—when faced with the prospect of a cheese plate, or a second bottle of that extremely good red . . . well, resistance is suddenly futile.

The problem is that everything around us—advertising, aromas, opinions—exerts a subtle pull on our behavior and our salivary glands. The food industry, driven by profit, wants us to eat. All the time. And it has spent a great deal of effort and money laying subtle traps to get our snouts in the trough. We all know about the freshly baked bread smells in supermarkets and how they lead you blindly to the checkout accompanied by cinnamon waffles and a quart of whipped cream—but the psychological manipulation goes deeper by far. You're more likely to buy a pastry in a shop that smells of coffee. People are known to order dessert in a restaurant simply because of the kind of music being played. And perhaps most bizarrely, we apparently spend more in a supermarket if we shop in a counterclockwise direction.

The best you can do is to plan ahead to resist the siren song of that fourth glass of Chardonnay, the sale on Hershey's Kisses, or the leftover baked ziti in the fridge. Over the next nine chapters, you'll equip yourself with hundreds of ways to do just that. For now, simply recognize temptation for what it is: temporal and transient. Breathe, move on, and it's gone. Feel strong. If a retail environment smells delicious, it's time to smell a rat. Oh, and shop backwards. Unleash your inner contrarian.

20 UNDERSTAND HUNGER

Many of us never give our bodies the chance to feel even the slightest bit empty, surfing as we do from one snack to the next. Research has found that many overweight people eat in response to all emotion, no matter what they feel. Hunger, it turns out, has little to do with it.[12]

At least once a day, then, try to put off eating until you feel hungry. Not ravenous, but more than just peckish. Experience real physical hunger, rather than a mild longing for lunch. Give your stomach the chance to growl at the postman—but don't, please, abstain utterly from food and drive yourself insane with cravings. Here's why: Scientists have found that ghrelin, a hormone that's produced in the stomach and that signals hunger to the brain, can make *all* food desirable. This may once have provided an adaptive advantage to humans, who needed to feast on any amount of garbage when times were lean. But now? Calamitous.

According to a report in the journal *Cell Metabolism*, ghrelin stimulates the same reward centers of the brain that have been linked to drug-seeking behavior.[13] Aha. This explains so much. Such as the popularity of hot dogs, spray cheese, and Pop Tarts, as well as why a bucket of divine, delicious, delectable fried chicken seems so appalling once you've demolished half of it and appeased the ghrelin gremlin. (As actress Beth McCollister puts it, "Food is like sex: when you abstain, even the worst stuff begins to look good.") Knowing this, you need to get a handle on your hunger, noticing it but keeping it comfortably at bay.

21 DRINK MORE WATER

It is an established tenet of dieting folklore that water will somehow miraculously facilitate weight loss—as if it gushes through your system seeking out fat cells as it goes, transporting them south like logs over Niagara. Alas, this is not the case.

There is, however, evidence to suggest that increasing water consumption will increase your metabolic rate (the rate at which calories are

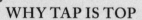

WHY TAP IS TOP

Americans spend $15 billion a year on bottled water, a product that boasts one of the highest markups in the known universe. Thanks to a gradual raising of eco-consciousness, however, ordering tap water is increasingly fashionable, and a good thing, too: It costs infinitely less than bottled. (For the finest taste, filter it and keep it in an earthenware or glass vessel in the fridge.)

Some of us, of course, still cherish the sass and security of the water bottle—its ease of availability, its portability, the subtle little signals it gives out. If tap water really doesn't float your boat, find a water that you do like; that way, you'll drink more of it. Personally, I have always been partial to Badoit and San Pellegrino because they have small, well-behaved bubbles and the kind of mineral content that appeals to me. Jennifer Aniston is said to prefer Fiji water, a rich source of silica (accounting, one would like to think, for her swishy hair and glowing skin). If you dine at the upscale Claridges Hotel in London, you'll be offered a Water Menu, featuring the superior 420 Volcanic for about $70 a liter—though you can, if you're both stingy and sensible, order a jug of tap water free of charge.

burned). A study from Berlin's Franz-Volhard Clinical Research Center found that subjects increased their metabolic rate by 30 percent after drinking about 17 ounces of water.[14] Increasing water consumption by 1.5 liters a day would burn an estimated additional 17,400 calories over the course of a year, equaling a weight loss of around 5 pounds.

American researchers have concluded that while there's no scientific reason to drink the "recommended" eight 8-ounce glasses of water a day, up to 75 percent of us *are* chronically dehydrated.[15] (A dry mouth is the last sign of dehydration, not the first.) There are other watertight reasons for drinking more fluids. Water fills your belly, for one, which is why so many people swear by drinking a glass before each meal. It also stops you from mistaking thirst for hunger. (According to the Watershed Wellness Center, 37 percent of people have a thirst mechanism so weak that they misinterpret it as hunger.) Drinking water keeps your mouth occupied when it would otherwise be anticipating a tasty donut. It's a natural appetite suppressant, and, though it won't wash fat cells away, it will flush out salts and toxins and other superfluous junk your body could do without. What's more, the University of Washington has shown that one simple glass of water before bed shuts down midnight hunger pangs for 100 percent of dieters.[16] That's some success rate, and all for the cost of a trip to the tap.

3

BODY BASICS

IT STARTS IN YOUR PANTS

With those first principles stashed under your belt, it's time to get down to the bottom line. A lack of body confidence means that we tend to cover everything up, hoping yards of fabric will camouflage us and hide the places where we wobble and jiggle. It won't, though. It will only make us look like a tent. A great body shape, in common with a great building, starts with reliable foundations. Your weight does not exist in limbo, some theoretical number that defines your very essence. Your weight is your whole body—all of it, from fingertips to eyelashes—and not just those love handles and hateful extra pounds that are getting you down. So you need to begin to nurture a positive vision of a whole new you. Think it, see it, and pretty soon you'll be it. Start at the ground floor and work your way up.

TA-DA! DO THE MOUNTAIN POSE

So you want to walk tall? Instead of parading up and down stairs with an encyclopedia balanced on your head, as advocated by Swiss finishing schools, try yoga. It is one of the best routes to flexibility, body consciousness, and refined posture. If your schedule is just too packed to allow a full session, try simply doing Mountain Pose, known in Sanskrit as Tadasana, for 5 minutes each morning. It can have a profound influence on your physical and mental well-being and improve your posture to no end. Here's how:

* Stand with your feet hip-width apart, toes spread.

* Distribute your weight evenly between your feet.

* Stand tall.

* Draw your shoulders back and down.

* Tuck your tailbone under.

* Keep your chin parallel to the floor and let your hands hang at your sides.

* Relax. Breathe. Be still.

Yoga manuals tend to say things like "allow your head to float upward off your shoulders," which is a crazy-sounding way of telling you to relax and let go. So try to clear your mind—it may be the only chance you have in your hectic day to do so. Stop thinking about what you're having for supper. Yes, the windows really do need cleaning. But this is your time. Be here, now.

22 PERFECT YOUR POSTURE

We're in the business of looking willowy, right? Lean? We're aiming to look less like a cinder block, more like a long, tall drink of water. Now think about an orangutan. Lovely creature, yes. Willowy, no. Giraffes are willowy.

You do not want to look as though your knuckles trail the floor when you walk. You want to give the impression that you could reach the highest leaves on the tallest tree, and this applies just as well to 5-foot-nothings as it does to 6-foot-somethings. The difference is all in your posture.

Interestingly, it is often tall women who have the worst posture, perhaps because they are self-conscious about their height. Others are embarrassed by their breasts, seeking to minimize them by hunching their shoulders and rounding their lower back. As a result, we end up with a paunchy tummy and a mild stoop, which does nothing at all for a cashmere sweater.

Good posture has all manner of beneficial effects. It means your skeleton is aligned, with your bones in the right places and not under undue stress. It will also make you look way better in a cocktail dress. So hold that head up high (this also helps with the double chin), pull in those abs, raise the rib cage, lengthen that neck, and away you go.

Clothes, incidentally, can have a significant effect on posture. A tight-fitting jacket and good shoes can change the way you stand and walk. If you've ever shuffled along like a flower child because you're wearing flip-flops, if you've ever stretched like a kitten while wearing mohair, if you've ever strutted like a CEO in a pantsuit, you'll recognize the truth in these words.

23 GET FITTED FOR A NEW BRA

As Kate Winslet says, "I start with the bra. If the bra's right, everything else falls into place." Don't you adore that? It sounds so utterly effortless that it makes you want to lie down on a couch and eat fudge. But Ms. Winslet is on to something. The right bra—by which I mean one that not only rises to the occasion (whether that's taking out the garbage or dancing till dawn), but also *fits*—is a dieter's dream.

A properly fitted bra will treat your entire body to an instant upgrade. It will improve your posture (see page 49), streamline your silhouette, separate your bosom from your waist, draw the eye away from your stomach, and fool onlookers into thinking you've lost either 5 pounds or 5 years. It could well be the best $40 you'll ever spend.

The issue, though, is that so few of us *are* wearing the right bra. The lingerie industry estimates that 70 percent of American women are wearing the wrong size right now.[1] Breasts are brilliant—ask anyone—and yet we routinely house them in a garment that amounts to little more than an afterthought, as if we're stashing them there for safekeeping until we might need them. Are you perhaps ladled into a cup too small, so that you threaten to spill over like a tremulous soufflé? Do you have four breasts, courtesy of a badly fitted bra? Do you identify with P. G. Wodehouse's description: "She looked as if she had been poured into her clothes and had forgotten to say 'when'"?[2]

If so, it's time to come to grips with your boobs. I did this myself not long ago, by visiting the renowned rooms of a high-end lingerie house in London, home of all that is fitting in brassieres and purveyor of undergarments to the Queen. Her Majesty gazes down from a photograph behind the cash register, superbly contained in foundation garments and royal regalia, her chest somehow staunch and dependable, the very manifestation of the British monarchy. I arrived a size 36C and, after a rather intimate moment in a dressing room with a delightful woman named Gina, I emerged a 30E. I was astonished. You could have knocked me over with a feather. And it all happened in a flash. Gina took one look at my naked back and knew that I had been roaming the land for decades saddled with the wrong bra. Within seconds I was eased into a bra that was both substantially bigger (in the cup) and substantially smaller (in the band) than I had been wearing for ages. This, it transpires, is the classic error and one that is simplicity itself to fix. The result? Things were certainly looking up. I'd gone from droop to boop—and all because the bra was doing the work. Oprah, it turns out, was dead right when she promised "Every woman watching, this is going to change your life. Everyone's talking about it. And I'm revealing a beauty secret that literally performs miracles. It can reverse aging. It can make you look 10, even 20 pounds lighter." Yes, a well-fitted bra is a miracle indeed. I strolled out onto the street and a construction worker shouted "great knockers!" at me from his scaffolding. I would have tossed an offended "stupid jerk!" in his direction if I hadn't been busy feeling quite so pleased with myself.

YOUR GUIDE TO BRA BRILLIANCE

* Bras, like men, lose their potency over time, so get fitted for a new bra every 6 months, treating it like a trip to the dentist (but cheaper and way more fun).

* Take your time choosing a bra. Why hurry? This is worth 3 months at the gym. (Or 6 weeks on the Cabbage Soup Diet.)

* Once you and a professional have determined the correct size, lean forward into the bra. Run two fingers between breast and cup to ease everything into position, and adjust the straps—you want them firm but friendly.

* If the back band rides up, your bra is too big.

* Buy a bra that feels snug on its loosest hook setting; it will stretch with every wash.

* Your breasts should completely fill the cups, but not overspill.

* If you have four boobs where there should be two, your cup is too small.

* Larger cup sizes need an underwire for added support; it should lie flat against your breastbone.

* Raise your arms. Your bra should stay put.

* If a bra fits well, it shouldn't pinch or poke or hassle you at parties.

* Check your bra by standing up straight—the center of your bust should fall halfway between your elbow and your shoulder. If it's south of the equator, you need to hike it all back up.

* If you require assistance in the oomf department, technology has recently stepped right up: try Fashion First Aid's range of Boostits, Liftits, Concealits, and Tapeits—a series of clever products that will perk up your chest, keep it under control, or conceal pushy nipples. (Visit usefulchickstuff.com.) As an added bonus, once removed and rolled around in the palm of the hand, a Boostit apparently makes a very satisfying stress ball.

And so my new breasts and I have been out and about, meeting and greeting. My husband is delighted with this turn of events and has taken to buying me a new wardrobe of bras to cope with this Barbie to whom, it turns out, he is married. So, all in all, everyone's a winner.

Interestingly, over the past decade alone, the average U.S. bra size has increased from 34B in 1985 to 36C today.[3] If your own cup runneth over, go to brasmyth.com, which caters to women from AA to H. Either way, it's well worth going to a professional to be fitted; most stores tend to give you a cursory once-over and a flick of a tape measure, sending you off to the register with the word "average" stamped on your forehead. Specialists like Gina are, by contrast, trained in the art of the bra, and you'll be surprised by how far off-target your current effort is. According to Gina and her co-workers, we ought to be fitted every time we buy a bra. Changing hormone levels, the Pill, your diet, and weight changes will all affect your bust size; it will almost certainly fluctuate, even in the relatively short term, so it's best to keep abreast of your chest.

24. RECOGNIZE THE IMPORTANCE OF PANTIES

Gosh, don't you just know when you've got it wrong? Who hasn't experienced the discomfort of the wedgie—that impish slice of thong lodged between your cheeks, insinuating itself as you saunter down the street? You wiggle. You do a little two-step. You launch into the Charleston, but to no avail. Eventually—oh rats—you just *have* to stop and pluck it out, hoping that bystanders won't notice that you're adjusting your panties.

Or how about those panties with the elastic just a *smidge* too tight, the ones that leave a welt of smarting red across your belly and your thighs in danger of losing their blood supply? Or the ones where the elastic has completely given up, so that you are oddly vulnerable of losing them entirely . . . the ones where there's way too much going on and your silhouette has to cope with ribbons, ruffles, lacing, pockets, and witty one-liners scrawled across your bum . . . the ones that clutch at your buttocks in too-intimate a manner, as if testing for ripeness, leaving you with a vicious case of Visible Panty Line. (Nothing, incidentally, adds pounds like VPL.)

Of course, no 21st-century woman should suffer in this way; the advent of proper underwear ought to have wiped it out at about the same time that smallpox disappeared from the world stage. But still, there are so many ways to get your knickers in a twist. Few items in your wardrobe have such a huge impact—not only on your shape and your look, but also on your day. The wrong underpants can put you off your game, lose you a tennis match, make you snap at your partner, prohibit potentially delightful sexual encounters, and generally be ruinous to your well-being.

As you may surmise, I have spent the better part of my career charting the ups and downs of women's panties. I lived, on behalf of *you*, dear reader, through the startling goosing of Donna Karan's "body" in the eighties, the aggressive G-strings of the nineties, and finally the roomy comfort of maternity underpants, built to house a family of four and still leave room for a chocolate éclair. I have done big bloomers and tiny tangas, I've gone frou-frou, sporty, and commando. And what I have learned from this odyssey can be distilled into a quartet of Panty Regulations that you'd do well to heed.

1. **A thong is a glorious thing.** It is nearly not a panty at all, more the *idea* of a panty, making it the ideal partner for all manner of pants, particularly those clingy ones that demand that your underwear should take a backseat. G-strings may be less fashionable than in their heyday (when Alexander McQueen invented low-cut "hipster" pants and we all, in a fit of collective hysteria, decided the crack was immensely cool). But you still need a handful in your arsenal if you are to triumph in very demanding clothes.

2. **Boy shorts will do the rest.** The cut is gracious to the lower curve of a bottom, which means it does the job of a G-string without the discomfort and with a bit more decorum.

3. **Fancy panties are great on a date,** but they're not worth a whole lot if you're looking for a smooth, lean line. They are, however, a superior shortcut to improving mood and body image (see Step 29).

4. **Seamless underwear.** They work beautifully, and they feel like a treat, too—not a saucy, *ooh-la-la* treat, but a private, practical one. Seamless underwear is ideal beneath unforgiving pants—anything

in white, anything with a high waist, anything with a jersey cling. Calvin Klein makes several varieties of these undies, as do Victoria's Secret and The Gap.

25 SHIFT YOUR SHAPE WITH SOLUTION LINGERIE

If you want to create the illusion of a flawless silhouette (and who doesn't?), you really need to put your underwear to work. Next time you're in nothing but your unmentionables, do a little dance in front of the mirror. If you're all wobble and jiggle where you'd like to be taut and toned, get with the program and invest in these mighty beasts. Don't, though, be dismayed when you unroll your new "shapewear." This is not about sex, it's about shape. I suggest that you introduce yourself in private. You'll be confronted with a salami-skin of Lycra that promises to smooth your groove and send you out into the waiting world with a figure to make grown men whimper.

What's odd is that these undergarments are *massive*—both in size and in popularity. It all started a decade or more ago on the red carpet, when stars were poured into foundation garments by their canny stylists, who well knew the insatiable curiosity of the paparazzi lens. Soon, we were all at it. Hey, if Jessica Alba, Carmen Electra, and Halle Berry could do it, we thought, then why not us?

Along came Spanx: revolutionary control-top pantyhose designed to contain all your wobbly bits and bearing the slogan "Don't worry, we've got your butt covered!" A revolution ensued. They are, I'm reliably told, the undergarment of choice for Diane Sawyer, Hillary Clinton, Susan Sarandon, and Joan Rivers. Renee Zellweger apparently "flipped out over them" when they first appeared in 2000, and Oprah Winfrey still rarely takes hers off. Why? These über-underpants, which, in certain formats, stretch from knee to bust, really do contain you like no other. Cleverly, they manage this feat of engineering without the excess blubber escaping at some other inopportune point (such as at the wrist).

THE WHAT AND WHERE OF SHAPEWEAR

The issue today certainly isn't a lack of options. If anything, it's the sheer wealth of stealth-wear out there that can confuse a girl. What used to be a simple stroll around the lingerie department at your local store has turned into an all-out battle of the bulge. You can, should you wish, purchase a Hi-Waist Thigh Trimmer, a Deep Plunge Body Suit, a Sculpted Bottom Boyleg . . . or perhaps a Super Smoother, a Waist Cincher, a Body Briefer, a Tummy Tamer, and, yes, good old Magic Pants.

These days, it's all about technology. There's money in them there hills, which means that there is an awful lot of R&D going on behind the scenes, producing ever more effective underthings. Very soon, we should be able to slap on a Super Slimmer and disappear almost entirely, leaving our date to pick up the tab.

One reason for the runaway success of "solution lingerie" is that it allows women to wear all manner of fashion, no matter how revealing or inadvisable. If you're plunging at the front and back, splitting to the thigh and shearing to the tush, there's not a whole lot of places for a body to hide. Today, there is bound to be a shape-shifter just for you. Some, when worn alone, will make you look like Ethel Merman; others, more like Lance Armstrong. You'll just have to suck it in and see which works for you.

Your only task in all of this is to ascertain precisely where your body needs the most help, and then buy accordingly. As a rule, it's best to purchase in person rather than online; these things need a body to bring them to life. If you really can't get to your nearest department store for a comprehensive fitting session, go to

These garments appeal not only because they do what they say they will, but also, I suspect, because they are a million miles from the sturdy panty girdles that you may have seen your grandmother roll on (a sight that probably stayed with you long after she was figleaves.com, a great Web site that stocks fantastic undergarments.

You'll notice that the latest innovations take inspiration from plastic surgery techniques, using knitted elastic of differing weights, stretchiness, and strength to echo the cuts a surgeon might make to flatten the stomach, smooth the thighs, or lift the buttocks. The upshot is an intelligent foundation garment, one that knows where to hold tight and where to relax, where to redistribute excess and where to let it loose—which scores the wearer a little more comfort and a good deal more confidence when exiting a taxi. Unsurprisingly, the company that specializes in just such a product (Dr. Rey's Shapewear) sold $1.5 million worth of shapewear in its first weekend of sales.

My personal favorite, given my own soft spots, is the Yummie Tummie—a series of tanks and tees designed by Heather Thomson, a fashion associate of Beyoncé and Jennifer Lopez. The tops, available at yummietummie.com, feature a midsection that holds in a belly and minimizes muffin top. "The effects of Yummie Tummie are dramatic for the wearer, both physically and mentally," says Thomson. Well, hallelujah! Ideal for a woman like me, who would gladly sell her belly on eBay, or even swap it for an interesting set of spoons.

Whatever garment you choose—the "skincarewear," perhaps, or the strapless body reducer—you're bound to shave off a few pounds, and all for the cost of a new pair of shoes. You'd be a fool not to. As if to clinch the deal, we're now starting to see the arrival of shapewear for men, including slimming girdles. The *Wall Street Journal* has reported on the burgeoning market for "support boxers" to lift and firm the backside and "waist eliminators" to tame the gut. If your man wears a mirdle, then surely you should, too?

gone). My own grandmother would take hours to hoist and shoehorn herself into the confines of a rubberized foundation garment, assisted by a liberal dusting of talcum powder and a very forgiving husband.

My how times have changed. I wore mine just this morning, and I can tell you, they're unbeatable if you want to look lithe and lovely as you go about your daily business. You wouldn't want to wear them if you were in line for a saucy rendezvous, mind you. But for times when it's all look and no touch? No contest.

26 LEARN HOW TO WALK WELL

As dear, dear Sir Laurence Olivier once declared, "Give me the shoes and I've got the part!" Heaven knows, some of us need all the help we can get. I hate to carp, but British women seem peculiarly afflicted with poor gait, our feet slapping on the moist pavement as if there's bound to be bad news just around the corner. Worse, just watch most British brides as they galumph down the aisle in their 1,000-pound frocks and dainty satin mules. My friend Josephine walked to the altar like the front half of a Clydesdale, which rather ruined the effect of her Vera Wang. And it's not just the Brits; plenty of American women plod rather than walk, as if carrying the weight of the world.

Mastering the gentle art of walking is a simple task that can carve the appearance of weight from a hunched and folded frame. I recommend walking lessons to anyone who has ever fallen downstairs into a party of new work colleagues gathered in a basement bar (me), anyone who has fallen *upstairs* while carrying hot chocolate (me), and anyone who regularly wears odd shoes (not "odd" as in "mismatched," but "odd" as in "inappropriate"—again, *me*).

Here is a tip-top lesson in how to walk gracefully, courtesy of the marvelous Jean Broke-Smith (former principal of the Lucie Clayton school of grooming and modeling): Stand up tall, clench your derriere, and move forward with your heels following a line along the floor and your toes pointed out just a bit. Place one foot in front of the other, then gracefully transfer your weight onto the heel of the front foot, then through the foot and onto the toe; as you pick up the back foot, place it in front. Repeat until you get where you're going. The idea is that you glide, with poise and balance (and with, I'm told, Jean's voice chanting "heel-instep-toe, heel-instep-toe" in your head).

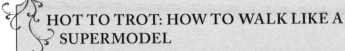

HOT TO TROT: HOW TO WALK LIKE A SUPERMODEL

Though you still see the occasional half-gallop down the runway, most models know how to walk well, a talent honed through years of practice. As model Jessica Stam says, "First impressions are a big deal, whether you're walking up to the podium to give a presentation or into a restaurant for a blind date . . . When a woman walks more confidently, it can really affect the way other people see her—and the way she feels about herself." If you've ever watched Naomi Campbell's sashay or Gisele Bündchen's confident stomp, you'll know what Stam is getting at. Here's how to do it their way, for those days when you want to take a room by storm.

* Keep your shoulders back and down, head straight, chin up, eyes focused gently at middle distance.

* Tilt your pelvis forward a little. Not too much, or you will topple over backward and land in a lap.

* Place the *ball* of your foot down first, not the heel. Think prima ballerina, and point away.

* Face your toes forward. One foot is placed in line with the next, so your footprints would make a straight line in the sand. You are not a duck, so don't waddle.

* Take longish strides, raising your whole foot off the ground as you go.

* Engage your abs to stabilize yourself, then relax at the hip. Do this, and you'll manage all manner of frivolous shoes like a pro.

27 BUY A CORSET

In my hometown of Brighton, England, down a suitably Dickensian alley, is the She Said Erotic Boutique, a crooked little shop that's home to a fetching collection of ostrich feathers, silken brassieres, and sexy underwear. The shop assistants all have tiny waists, wild-cherry lips, and cute, choppy bangs. They're true mistresses of the burlesque and are all experts at making a woman—any woman—come over all drop-dead *femme fatale*. One visit and you're guaranteed to drop a dress size, simply by discovering the incomparable power of the corset. Victoria Beckham has known this for years. Kylie Minogue, too. So what's keeping you?

I went to She Said recently and bought a corset, a golden satin number with black lace trim and eight wicked garters. It was called the "Moulin Rouge," cost over $200, and once I'd been maneuvered into it, there I was: all bosom, all curvy, all 22 inches of waist. After years of griping about the abomination of corsetry and any other contraption that turns women into dolls and men into dogs, it was here that I had my Damascene conversion. I was Madame de Pompadour, or maybe Scarlett Johansson on a flight of scarlet stairs. An hourglass figure, I told my reflection in the mirror, is just sensational. It graces a body with curves and swoops, and spoons a chest into position like a couple of scoops of vanilla ice cream. Who would willingly turn that down?

The flirtatious interplay of enhanced bosom, contained tummy, and diminished waist is of course pure female, a truth recognized throughout history. Consider the iconic images of womankind, and you'll see that the waist almost always plays a starring role. *The Rokeby Venus* by Velásquez. *The Swing* by Fragonard. Scarlett O'Hara clutching the bedpost as she's drawn into her corset. Dior's New Look. Monroe, Mansfield, Madonna . . . the picture is constant: an erotic conflation of billowing skirts and a minuscule, embrace-me waist.

According to our long-established socio-cultural norms, women ought to nip in at the equator. Indeed, at the end of the 19th century, a girl's eligibility was judged by the size of her waist—which should be "twice the circumference of her neck, which, in turn, should be twice the circumference of her wrist," as defined by the dressmakers' guidelines of the day. If you were to ask a social anthropologist, they'd explain that the imagery is so consistent because there is an evolutionary imperative at play. The "magic ratio" of waist to hips is, for women, 7:10. "That silhouette is going to have a sexual appeal at a primeval level," argued author Desmond Morris long ago. "It's signaling the child-bearing pelvic girdle, there's no great mystery about that."

Though we are, as a gender, tending toward a thickening of the waist over time, there is no reason I can see that you shouldn't enhance your assets with a little artifice. You can buy a corset in several types of shops, of course, but I would advise you to go to a specialist corsetiere (Google will direct you to your nearest)—if only for the thrilling experience of being laced into this peculiar contraption by a proper professional with choppy bangs. You won't want to wear it to go grocery shopping or pick up the kids from school, but for those big, razzle-dazzle moments in a girl's life, nothing can quite match it. Wear your corset under your clothes, a clandestine thrill, or out and proud over a sleek shirt. Either way, it will snatch away several pounds and stow them somewhere unknown, out of sight.

28 KNOW THE POWER OF BLACK OPAQUE TIGHTS AND WHY THEY SIMPLY LOVE YOUR LEGS

Opaque tights are truly a gift from heaven. They are central to our existence, one of the 10 vital inventions since the dawn of time (others include Superglue, tweezers, Maybelline mascara, fire, wheels, ear plugs, and Manolo Blahnik). Back in the eighties, when my young legs were rarely out of them, opaques possessed the indefinable talent of making your shins and ankles, your calves, and even your knees look slimmer. They did this without dieting or scandalously priced body-firming creams. They did it without fuss, without nudging you in the ribs and saying "Hey, you have *got to* check this out!" They just did it as a matter of course, nonchalantly, as if clothes performed this kind of miracle all the time.

On top of these great gifts to womankind, opaque tights concealed a multitude of sins, from knobby knees to ingrown hairs, from cracked heels to pasty legs, from scraped shins to unintentional exposure of that bit on the back of your upper thigh that you never, ever get to see yourself unless you are very committed to yoga. Beyond all this, opaque tights were warm! They were comfortable! They came in all manner of weights—and the thick ones lasted for months. What more could you want?

Well, not much—apart from the promise that these wonder hose should be in fashion *always*. Sadly, this was not to be. Opaque tights, like cowboy boots, are trapped forever in the revolving door of fashion—sometimes emerging on the cool side to strut about, making a miniskirt look like dynamite and you look like one of Robert Palmer's guitar girls from the "Addicted to Love" video. And then, just as you're feeling confident that your legs will never again look so *wow*, opaques swing over to the other side, cast off and blackballed by all but the most hopeless dressers.

The replacement, generally, is patterned tights, which—by some fascinating precept of style—manage to have precisely the opposite effect. I have never met a woman (nor a man, come to think of it), whose legs are enhanced by fussy hosiery. Fishnets, yes. In fact, fishnets, fabulous. Seamed stockings? Of course. (Few optical tricks will elongate a leg like a dark line heading north.) But on no account should we indulge in white tights, unless we are playing the lead in a production of Peter Pan. No Pucci swirls, no rococo curlicues, no witty squiggles. Chevrons, spots, lace, and rainbow stripes should similarly be reserved for the under-five set, and even then I'd err on the side of caution. Instead, I suggest we all wear black opaques, regularly, persistently, as often as we wear jeans. Often enough that people notice and think, "Hey, would you look at that? Opaques are back! It's fine to continue wearing mine." This, my friends, is fashion democracy in action.

29 PUT ON YOUR BEST UNDERWEAR; DON'T SAVE IT

I know women who have an entire collection of lingerie that they are "saving for a special occasion." These superb frillies lie neatly folded, in a dark drawer or on a distant shelf, in tissue wrap or a muslin bag, while the everyday drones of the underwear drawer—those bikinis, briefs, and bras in much-washed cotton—go about their duties. The really good stuff comes out to play only once in a very long while, on special occasions and holidays and evenings when there's the genuine prospect that they'll see action—from a lover, perhaps, or a competitive friend.

Admit it. When was the last time you wore that push-up bra in golden satin? The adorable set in coffee-colored lace? The sugar-pink cami with the mocha ribbon lacing? Though we're buying ever more of the stuff, most of the time—because we're in a rush or in a rut—we don't wear gossamer panties and woo-hoo bras. We stick instead to what we know best. This generally boils down to routine stock in a neutral color, worn in the earnest hope that we won't get hit by a bus or picked up by a stranger or find ourselves in a position where suddenly we have to show our panties in public (while getting changed at a spa, say, or falling off a bucking bronco at a barn dance). I was at a school sports day just this week, and I found myself jumping up and down as my son came in fourth in the sack race. "Nice panties," my great friend Lou whispered in my ear. And thank heavens it was Lou, for these panties were not nice. They were as old as the hills and might even have had the word "Wednesday" printed on the front, though it had long since faded away in the wash. It's possible I wore these panties my first semester in college, or for my driving test, or on the lap of a man named Keith whom I might have married if only he hadn't been named Keith. A good 20 years down the line, and the panties are still desperately clinging to life, cheering my boy on as he jumps through the heat of a summer's afternoon.

So, I well understand the reasons for playing it safe. Old panties are comfy panties. Reliable. My friend Nicky swears by several pairs that boast more than the regulation three holes, arguing that they have been with her through thick and thin and feel like dear old friends. Besides, silk underwear requires special washing procedures. (And leopard-print bras can feel a bit provocative for a 9 a.m. breakfast meeting with your accountant.) But . . . there is nothing quite so delightful, so indulgent, as wearing a flimsy, vulnerable nothing in whispering satin, a silk flower budding at the cleavage. Though I don't expect you to get dolled up like a box of truffles every single day, it is worth rolling out the good stuff on a fairly regular basis. Why? Psychology, stupid. If you treat yourself, you'll love yourself. You'll feel good about you, at an intimate, personal, mildly saucy level. Dressing as though you're expecting rain will influence the mood of your day. Dress like a goddess—even underneath that workaday navy pantsuit—and you just see what it does for your self-image. You may even find yourself having more sex. This, needless to say, is a very good thing. (See Step 86.)

4

HOW TO EAT PETITE, PART I

WHAT TO PUT ON YOUR FORK

Now that you've hit Chapter 4, you're probably feeling a little peckish. It's way past snack time, right? Mercifully, there are easy, healthy ways to eat that keep one eye on moderation and the other on the scale. What you need is consciousness. Awareness. A bit of Zen. Think before you drink, look before you eat. You don't need to make a song and dance out of it—just be conscious of your intake. It's the smart, sustainable method of controlling calories, and it sure beats dieting.

30 GET FRESH AND FEEL THE FORCE

If your idea of a balanced diet is a cookie in each hand, it's clearly time to reset your dial. Plenty of people—whether 90-pound waifs or 250-pound whoppers—are malnourished because they fail to eat sufficiently nutritious food. If you want to feel great and look incredible, you have to eat well, which means a varied diet with plenty of fresh fruits and veggies. Not exactly a shocking revelation, I know, but one worth repeating. So put down those cookies and climb on board. Here are six surefire ways to increase your vitamin content.

* **Eat in season—and locally.** If you suspect—as many do—that modern crop-breeding, accelerated growth, prolonged storage, and long-distance transport lower the nutritional value of food. So stand on your doorstep. Try to eat things from within a 25-mile radius; if you're in a vast metropolis, make it 40 miles, and pamper yourself with the knowledge that you're doing the planet a favor, too. A little investigation should yield a prodigious harvest, wherever you live.

  If I lived in the Bay Area of California, for example, I could eat sweet Bing cherries and syrupy Blenheim apricots from Brentwood, and heirloom tomatoes, clementines, and clams from Marin County. I'd stop off at the roadside for wild arugula, nettles, and watercress—as well as dragon fruit, pluots, goumi, and goji berries—all of it growing right there on my doorstep.

  Eating in this honest, grounded way may leave you feeling like a heroine in a Thomas Hardy novel, but let's be frank: Fitting this sort of eating into a busy life is undoubtedly a challenge. I recently spent an entire weekend picking blackberries from nearby fields and turning them into jelly; at 10 p.m. on Sunday night, I realized we hadn't had any *lunch* and the kids' school clothes were still trapped in the laundry basket nursing last week's grass stains. Clearly, we can't all spend limitless hours driving around the countryside to procure free-range sausages, we can't all know the family tree of the apples in our bowl. But we can make a stab at eating seasonally. Strawberries in December, as everyone knows, should be shot on sight. If your asparagus comes from Peru and you don't, it's time to alter your eating habits.

✳ **Uncook! Go raw!** You'll lose weight, for sure. This is, of course, fabulous news for hopeless cooks across the land. The idea is that nothing should be heated beyond 118°F (the point at which vitamins and vitality are lost). As David Wolfe, America's leading raw food guru, puts it: "The psychedelic feeling of pure joy that one derives from eating high-quality raw foods cannot be compared to anything one has experienced before. . . . Inner cleanliness is an exquisite feeling! On top of this, raw plant food gives you superhuman powers!" All that from alfalfa sprouts!

My dear friend Pen swears by the mystic power of her Shredded Beet Salad. It may not sound very exciting, but trust me when I tell you that it is sublime.

• For four people, roughly grate three medium-size fresh beets. Just scrub them under water, and don't bother peeling; it must be rough, or the beets will become slushy.

• Grate three carrots using the same large holes on your grater.

• Add one-quarter of a stalk of celery if you feel like it, or some grated apple.

• Mix the following to make a dressing:

    2 tablespoons horseradish

    2 tablespoons olive oil

    1 tablespoon freshly squeezed lemon or orange juice

    1 teaspoon spicy yellow mustard

    A garlic clove or two, diced, chopped, squashed—or not at all, if you are about to go on a date

    Salt and pepper to taste

• Dress the grated veggies and top with sesame or pumpkin seeds.

If you want some protein with that, give *crudo* a go; it's an Italian version of sushi. The tissue-thin raw fish—bass, bream, mackerel—is served with olive oil, lemon, and fresh herbs (rather than wasabi, soy sauce, and a shaving of pickled ginger).

* **Have it handy.** If you're a bit like Bree Van de Kamp, keep a selection of precut, crunchy crudités in iced water in the fridge. If you're a bit like me, buy the precut bags in the refrigerated produce section of your supermarket and tear them open as you need them. And keep fruit readily available, looking charming in a bowl, not exhausted beyond resuscitation in the crisper. Pears, as Eddie Izzard has noted, are particularly terrible in this respect: "They're gorgeous little beasts, but they're ripe for *half an hour*, and you're never there. They're like a rock, or they're mush . . . you put them in the bowl at home, and they sit there, going, 'No! No! Don't ripen yet, don't ripen yet. Wait till he goes out the room! Ripen! *Now now now!*'" It may be worth persevering with pears, though, watching them like a hawk for that brief moment of perfection: Researchers at the State University of Rio de Janeiro have found that overweight women who ate three small pears a day lost more weight on a low-calorie diet than women who didn't add fruit to their diet.[1]

* **Buy good, green, fresh herbs—not dried ones.** And while you're at it, keep olive oil in an airtight, opaque container to keep it vital and vibrant.

* **Think healthy.** In the past, I have always found crunchy health-food stores to be a mild turnoff. I only needed to stand in the aisles to be plagued with guilt. "I'm not worthy," my soul would yell. "I didn't recycle the honey jar." My leather shoes would step over the threshold and shout their provenance and price. "We're dead cows!" they'd shriek, "Expensive dead cows!" Mercifully, I have since matured and gotten over it—partly because, thanks to the eco revolution, the shops themselves have stepped out of the seventies and into the new millennium. If you're not doing it already, it's well worth taking a regular weekly spin around your local health-food store to see what grabs your attention—an aloe drink, perhaps, or a stick of all-natural licorice. Whatever keeps you off factory food is fine by me.

* **Know that calcium counts.** Though dairy has long been the demon in the fridge for dieters, it turns out that calcium—one of milk's vital components—can help facilitate weight loss. In studies, people on a

reduced-calorie diet who included some dairy foods lost significantly more weight than those who ate a low-dairy diet containing the same number of calories. Researchers at the University of Tennessee found that when fat cells are exposed to a calcium-rich environment, they break down more swiftly than they do in calcium-depleted conditions.[2] If you want to boost your calcium intake without resorting to the fat-fest that is Cheddar cheese, go for the brilliance of broccoli. It is high in vitamin C, too, which helps foster calcium absorption. And on those days when you're in a hurry, consider taking a calcium supplement.

31 EAT MORE SOUP

This is a stunningly simple way to eat less and still get a warm, full feeling in your belly. Soup, according to research from Penn State University, is a great appetite suppressant because it consists of a hunger-busting combination of liquids and solids.[3] Simply eat it before a meal (in the traditional way) and you can lower your overall calorie intake by up to 20 percent (compared to a meal without soup).

But there's more. Having a wholesome, humble soup for lunch rather than buying your usual sandwich could have an even more dramatic effect on your waistline. Many of the flamboyant sandwiches on sale in popular chains—the ones that look as if they could do a backflip, make a coin appear from your cleavage, and deliver a witty punch line—contain fiercely high levels of fat and salt, and the calories to match. Panera's Chicken Caesar Sandwich on Focaccia, which sounds wholesome and healthy, clocks in at 860 calories. A Big Mac, by contrast, contains 495 calories. Go figure.

You do need to be eating the right kind of soup, though. Some years ago, I decided to take the soup idea to the extreme by ditching lunch completely and replacing it with a tasty Cup-a-Soup instead. My favorite Chicken and Mushroom flavor, which I consumed for 2 weeks straight, contained 1.7 percent mushroom and 1.1 percent chicken—less than its content of monopotassium phosphate (an acidity regulator), and less still than E471 (an emulsifier). This, I soon found, was not a satisfying midday meal. By 3 p.m. I would be ready to gnaw the door. (Luckily, I generally had a bag of gummi bears on hand.) Hopeless. The Cabbage Soup Diet is similarly vile, about as appetizing as a warm fish milk shake, and—given its vicious odor and gas-promoting properties—a startlingly effective way to lose friends and alienate people.

What you really need is an honest, *nourishing* soup, preferably with some protein in it. (Beans and lentils will do the trick.) In a perfect world, you'd probably make your own, having first produced a fine stock from heritage vegetables grown in your garden. I am honestly thrilled for you if you inhabit such a world, but if not, the premises-made soups you find in delis and grocery stores come in a decent second. Look on the label to see how heavy it really is. As a rule cheesy soups, "cream-of" soups, and meat-fest soups are full of gratuitous calories and don't hold a candle to veggie broths (at least for our purposes). Go for delicate infusions—perhaps a Vietnamese Pho, with a kick of chili peppers, a fling of noodles, and masses of coriander. Try borscht, consommé, or miso (chock-full of essential amino acids, vitamins, and minerals) over chowder, bisque, and potage. If you have to use a knife and fork, you've lost the advantages that make soup your friend.

If you're going to make it yourself, soups demand a pleasing seasonal approach and are a great destination for leftovers. Improvise—though please don't do what my husband once did and produce "Roast Lunch Soup," using every last remaining scrap from Sunday's dinner, liquefied in a blender. Do, however, play. Chuck an egg and some minuscule quadretti pasta into well-seasoned, densely flavored chicken stock to make "pasta in brodo," a low-key, fun-filled favorite of my childhood. Root around in the bottom of the fridge for forgotten vegetables—the leftover butternut squash, the about-to-sprout potatoes, a few tired carrots. Boil them in the stock, throw in any handy herbs and a scattering of chili flakes, then blend and devour. Heaven in a bowl, and it will never taste the same twice (which is so much more than can be said of a Big Mac or a Starbucks muffin, both of which taste identical worldwide, regardless of your location).

Avoid serving with a hunk of bread or croutons or crackers (or Gruyère, aioli, or dumplings). But you knew that already. In summer, make it cool

SLUUURP! HOW TO EAT SOUP IN POLITE COMPANY

* Spoon in a gentle motion away from the table's edge.

* Fill your spoon three-quarters full.

* Scrape excess from the base of your spoon using the edge of the bowl.

* Turn to your right and enter into engaging conversation with any visiting dignitaries who might be seated there.

* Don't blow. Wait for the soup to cool in its own time.

* Do not put the entire spoon in your mouth; drink from the side of your spoon instead.

* Ssshh! Not so loud.

* You may, if you wish, tilt the bowl away from you to scoop up the dregs, but don't do this more than twice or you will seem ungraciously ravenous, like Oliver or Tiny Tim.

* Set your spoon down in the bowl between mouthfuls. Do not rest it on the tablecloth, where it will make a dreadful stain, for which the hostess may later bill you.

* When you're done, do not mop up with bread. What's done is done.

* Vogue's *Book of Etiquette*, by Millicent Fenwick, has the following to say about the final act: "When one has finished one's soup, the spoon is left in the soup plate, handle to the right, over the edge of the plate, parallel to the edge of the table; but it should never be left in a soup cup or any other cup. The spoon should lie on the saucer of the cup. Never, even for a moment, should a spoon be left sticking out of the cup."

* Ignore the above. Soup in a cup is a glorious thing, second only to hot chocolate in a mug, and should be enjoyed with abandon. Soup in a basket is less successful. Soup in a flask is, by the way, the perfect portable meal.

cucumber soup, green pea and mint, or zingy gazpacho. When cooking for friends, kick off a meal with a light brothy starter—it will fill you right up and ensure that you don't pig out when the main course rolls around.

As you dine, dwell upon the further evidence that you are doing yourself a whole lot of good: A 2-year French study of 5,000 individuals found that those who ate soup five or six times a week were more likely to have BMIs below 23 (that's lean), compared with those who infrequently or never ate soup, whose BMIs tended to be way up around 27.[4]

32 TAKE A NOTE FROM THE JAPANESE AND GET INTO RAW FISH. BETTER STILL, GO FISHING

You may already know that the Japanese have some of the lowest obesity rates in the developed world. While their traditionally low consumption of dairy is partly responsible for this enviable state of affairs, their diet also owes much to food served in varying degrees of rawness, keeping it nutritionally sound and engagingly natural. The other key difference is that the Japanese tend to consume a good deal less meat than Westerners do. According to the latest estimates, Japanese people eat about 99 pounds of meat per person per year. The annual figure in the United States is 286 pounds, while in France it's 227 pounds, and in Great Britain a still-substantial 180 pounds.[5] The average American eats less than one seafood meal each week, and that's usually fried.[6] What a shame. Fish is high in protein and low in saturated fat (unless you drown it in batter and fry it in a vat of oil). What's more, salmon, mackerel, eel—the oily fish—are admirably high in omega-3 essential fatty acids, which will help you with Sudoku when you are elderly.

As you might expect, raw fish retains the most nutrients. If you're going to try eating like the Japanese, go for sashimi over sushi (no rice!), and make sure it's as fresh as the morning breeze (it's amazing what the hot kiss of wasabi can do for a sliver of naked salmon). If, however, raw leaves you cold and you need a "cooked" flavor, try ceviche. The acid in the citrus marinade will "cook" the fish without heat, turning it from translucent to opaque before your very eyes. This is a traditional Latin

American method and requires (of course) the freshest fish you can muster. It works with bass, cod, and mackerel, but is particularly good with snapper, and even better eaten on the boat deck and accompanied by a very cold beer.

WHAT

1 red snapper fillet (or preferred fish) per person,
    boned, skinned, and cut into ½-inch cubes
Juice of 1 lime, juice of 1 lemon
Diced red onion (optional)
1 red chile pepper, seeded and finely chopped
A little salt, a grind of pepper, a hint of Tabasco to
    taste. (A suggestion of freshly grated ginger
    would be good, too.)

HOW

Place all ingredients in a glass or stainless steel bowl. Coarsely chop a fistful of coriander. Add, and eat within minutes (it only takes 2 minutes for the marinade to do its work), or put it in the fridge for a few hours, stirring very occasionally, or whenever you happen to be visiting for a beer.

There are caveats, though. Be aware of conflicting advice about the "safe" amount of fish to consume. While the Food and Drug Administration (FDA) recommends a limit of two portions of fish a week to avoid overexposure to potential pollutants, other health experts advocate three portions a week to maximize genuine health benefits. You should rely on your common sense to arrive at an amount that works best for you.

If you are more concerned about the sustainability issue, choose fish that have been certified by the Marine Stewardship Council, such as Pacific cod, hand-raked clams, Dover sole, Cornish sea bass, and so on. For the full lowdown, download the Marine Conservation Society's Good Fish Guide at fishonline.org.

If you want to find one excellent little fish that can address all of your needs, look to sardines: They're loaded with protein, high in omega-3s, cheap, and impressively low in contaminants, since they live low on the food chain. Go for sardines caught in traditional drift or ring nets and you've got yourself a very fine fish, especially if you brush them with herby, garlicky olive oil and grill them over searing hot coals.

33 BUY MORE FOOD THAT HAS NO LABEL

Make it a point to choose fresh, proper produce with a coating of earth, not shrink wrap. I know it's hardly a scoop to tell you that you'd do better to eat food as nature intended—but let's just say that I'm covering all bases here. If your potatoes are fries and your chicken is nuggets, not only are you doing your mouth a disservice, you're doing your waistline no good at all.

So go naked. It's apparently how Nicole Kidman maintains her enviable self. "She has healthy eating habits," says a friend. "She's very picky about what goes in her mouth—she doesn't eat anything from a box or a can." This should apply to most of what ends up in your shopping cart, and not only the fresh stuff. Products that don't require much in the way of packaging tend to contain fewer preservatives, additives, and synthetic chemicals. You could even make some of it yourself. (See the opposite page.)

34 RETRAIN YOUR PALATE, WAKE UP YOUR MOUTH

Fed up with your fridge? Jaded by the tedium of your kitchen cupboards? Does a shiftless apathy envelop you at the prospect of supper? Well, me too. Deciding what to cook, as anyone regularly saddled with that responsibility knows, is an abominable drag. Personally, I'm happy to shop, chop, cook, and clean up afterwards, and I may even throw in a song and dance routine—so long as someone tells me what to serve. There is no earthly point to wandering hopelessly around the supermarket sniffing for inspiration. You will emerge momentarily triumphant only to find that you have come home with a large

HOW VERY CULTURED: WHY DIY YOGURT IS SUBLIME

I don't want to freak you out, but what's to stop you from making your own yogurt? It's not beyond you, and yogurt is an all-round, calcium-rich, protein-fueled wonder-food—even though I stopped eating the stuff for a decade starting at age 8 because my friend Eddie Wall told me that yogurt was alive and, if you listened closely, you could hear it scream. I listened closely and spent my formative years with yogurt in my hair as a result. Never once heard it scream, though.

Before Eddie Wall ruined It, yogurt played a big part in my young life. One of my clearest childhood memories is of the leaf green Thermos my mother kept for the express purpose of making yogurt. It would sit on a windowsill, alive with promise, until time was up and she'd spoon out great quivering white dollops of fresh, cool, tangy deliciousness, easily as good as pudding (as long as you were allowed to add a slick of honey). While you can produce the stuff in a yogurt maker, the art of doing it in any old warm spot, in an old Thermos, is one that is well worth revisiting on a lazy rainy day. Here's what to do.

* Sterilize your milk (any milk, you choose) by heating to *near* boiling; stir to avoid scorching.

* Cool the milk by putting the pan in a sink half full of cold water.

* Stir in a couple of tablespoons of your groovy live culture. This can be any store-bought yogurt that boasts "active cultures" or—for greater reliability—use freeze-dried bacteria, available online or at the health-food store (where they now know you by name).

* Pour into a leaf green Thermos or similar airtight container.

* Let it incubate on a sunny window ledge for a day.

* Stick it in the fridge.

* Reserve enough to start your next batch. Use the starter within a week for best results.

* Adorn the rest with fresh raspberries, chopped hazelnuts, and a drizzle of—yes, go on then—honey.

pie and three different types of pasta. Better by far to know in advance at least some of the meals you're likely to consume over the next week or so.

Rather than rely on old standbys and faithful favorites, you'd do well to mix it up a bit. The Japanese, for instance, aim for five colors at each meal: red, blue-green, yellow, white, and black. Give it a go, and your vegetable intake will soar. Ancient Ayurveda, meanwhile, dictates that the key to a satisfying meal lies in the inclusion of all six basic tastes (sweet, sour, salty, bitter, pungent, and astringent). Nonsense? Perhaps. But a rounded, varied plate of food is bound to fill you and thrill you far more than a pizza, where every bite tastes broadly the same unless you happen upon a jalapeño. As a rule, if one food group covers your entire plate, you're on the wrong path.

Develop a loose repertoire of evening meals that are hasty, tasty, but above all low in fats and fast-release carbs. Write them down. Keep the list in your purse, not stuck to the fridge. (Who brings a fridge shopping?) Don't think of it as a menu plan, don't stick to it like glue, don't have it laminated and peer at it each morning, saying, "Ah, Tuesday! Must be tofu kebabs." But do think ahead, just a bit. When you are strolling around in your local supermarket, it helps to have a general idea of the kind of low-effort cooking that won't sink your ship.

Here are some of my favorites.

* **OK Fish.** I've always called it this because it hails from the kitchen of our friends the O'Kellys, who live in southern England, in the lea of the South Downs, surrounded by children and chickens. The idea is to chuck it all in the oven (the ingredients, not the children and the chickens, God forbid), Jamie Oliver style, and see what deliciousness emerges. It's different every time, and you have to be fond of olives right from the get-go, but OK Fish is always wholesome and hearty, cunningly dispensing with the usual carbo-loading brought on by your average British supper. So be a dear and don't ruin it all by mopping up the juices with a great hunk of bread.

WHAT

A packet of baby green beans (haricot verts),
   blanched in boiling water
A bunch of asparagus, blanched in boiling water
   (broccoli works, too)
Cherry tomatoes, some; chuck in the vine as well,
   for flavor
Greek olives—the black wizened ones, not kalamata
A good slosh of extra virgin olive oil
A lemon, squeezed (the rind goes in the pan, too)
Salmon—one fillet per person—seasoned with rock salt
   and coarse pepper
Chili flakes optional; herbs like coriander, thyme, or
   dill equally optional

HOW

Preheat your oven to 400°F. Put the veggies and
olives in a casserole dish, and place the seasoned fish
on top. Bake for 20 minutes, or until the fish is
cooked to your liking. Serve. Eat. Smile.

* **Tuna Fagioli.** This was one of the nonchalant little Italian suppers
I grew up on, when everyone else was having ham topped with
pineapple. These days, it seems to me to be the perfect supper—
comfortingly low in all the things you ought to avoid, but high in
boundless flavor. It is simplicity itself to prepare, a real pantry
standby, and—like chili con carne—it tastes even better on Day
Two. Use an excellent olive oil. (The price is your guide. Sorry, but
it is. Same goes for shoes—what do you want me to say?) The
classic fagioli uses cannellini beans, but you can mix and match.
Try kidney beans, black beans, whatever. I add a generous squeeze
of lemon juice to mine, together with a fistful of torn flat-leaf
parsley—not strictly the old-time Florentine recipe, but all the
more delicious for it.

WHAT

1 drained can of tuna (in water—no need to add
  second-rate oil to this dish)
2 cans of beans, drained
1 red onion, thinly sliced or chopped
Juice of half a lemon
1 crushed garlic clove
2 tablespoons (approximately) good olive oil
2 tablespoons white wine vinegar
A handful of flat-leaf parsley, torn
Rock salt and freshly ground pepper

HOW

Put everything in a bowl. Mix it up. Eat it, or stick it
in the fridge for later. Serve with juicy red tomatoes—
good ones that really taste tomatoey, as if they were
the distilled essence of a hot Tuscan day—quartered,
salted, olive-oiled—and quickly demolished.

What else? There are other great recipes that are right on the money in
terms of calories but are full of ramped-up flavor. You'll have your own
hit-list, but here are a few more of mine.

✳ **Oriental chicken salad.** Oven-cook four chicken breasts. Let them
  cool. Tear to shreds. Dress with a generous handful of coriander and
  mint leaves, chopped scallion, olive oil, 1 tablespoon of Thai fish
  sauce, 1 teaspoon of sesame oil, and the juice of 2 limes. Season and
  serve on a crunchy bed of iceberg lettuce and cucumber slices, dousing
  the lot with the remaining dressing.

✳ **Tuna Niçoise.** I boil baby new potatoes, eggs, and baby green beans
  (haricot verts) in the same saucepan. Once boiling, the beans come out
  on a slotted spoon after 5 minutes, the eggs after 10, and the potatoes
  after 15. Cool it all, with the hard-boiled eggs plunged into ice-cold water
  to keep the yolks from graying. Build a substantial nest of leaves dressed
  with lemon juice and olive oil (3 parts oil to one part juice) in a large bowl.
  Add cherry tomatoes; pumpkin, sunflower, sesame, or poppy seeds;

olives; and anchovies to taste. Then add the chilled beans, potatoes, and eggs (cut into quarters). Season tuna steaks (1 per serving) with salt and pepper. Sear the steaks for not more than a few minutes on a hot griddle. (You want the center to stay pink.) Squeeze the steaks with lemon as they cook, rest for 5 minutes, then place them precariously, deliciously, on the waiting salad. Add lemon wedges, coarse pepper, and a glitter of sea salt. Spectacular. Increase your bean-to-potato ratio to maximize the good stuff, or better still, skip the potatoes altogether; there's more than enough going on here without them. A can of tuna works perfectly well if you haven't got the fresh (and far more expensive) stuff.

✳ Beef carpaccio—raw and sliced ultra-thin—with arugula leaves. Good beef. Fresh greens. Lemon. Olive oil. The usual.

✳ Buffalo mozzarella, prosciutto, tomatoes (more of those tasty ones), and basil leaves drizzled with olive oil and high-quality balsamic vinegar.

✳ Smoked trout, shredded into low-fat crème fraîche. Add crunchy sliced celery and horseradish to taste, and serve with interesting greens. (A romaine, perhaps.)

✳ Omelet with chile peppers and onions, not cheese and ham.

✳ Grilled cod with steamed green vegetables. Sugar snaps, tender-stem broccoli, asparagus. All good.

✳ Smoked haddock with poached egg and a wilted heap of young spinach leaves. (Drain everything well on paper towels; your food should not float.)

✳ A whole baked fish—sea bass, say—with herbs in its belly and salsa verde on the side.

✳ Endive leaves with fresh pear and walnuts, spiked with a crumble of blue cheese.

✳ Award yourself small tastes of—oh, I don't know—pitted olives, coarse hummus, and fingers of whole wheat pita. Add a tang of feta cheese, a dollop of baba ghanoush, celery sticks, red pepper slices, baby carrots, and artichoke hearts. Or go Greek with the classic cucumber/tomato/red onion/feta combo, drizzled with extra virgin olive oil and a squeeze of lemon.

35 CHOOSE FAT-BURNERS, NOT FATS

Some foods demand that you eat more. They conspire and tease, they breed cravings and hankerings, they gaze at you from the open packet and invite you to have *just one more*. (We're only too familiar with "No one can eat just one," "Once you pop you can't stop," and "Betcha can't eat just one.") Thus ensnared, your blood sugar bounces around like a beach ball, and—bang—you're down to the last Pringle before you've had time to loosen your belt.

Other foods, by divine contrast, satisfy. They contain clever components that can stimulate a metabolism or rev up your day. These nutrient-rich foods are considered by many to be almost magical in their capacity to crush hunger and speed up your body's fat-burning power. Here, listed in no particular order, are nine flab-busting, fat-burning foods—and why they work. Don't panic. You don't need to eat them all at every meal. You are not Gwyneth Paltrow, and this is not a fad diet. But try to include them on your plate from time to time. Choose these at the expense of their less-effective brethren. And keep that belt tightened.

Grapefruit. No, no, no, *not* the Grapefruit Diet, which requires you to go about your daily business in the constant companionship of a couple of grapefruit, your only respite being the occasional pink one or perhaps a nice glass of juice. To depend so heavily on a single foodstuff is both dull and disastrous. But . . . there is some evidence to suggest that grapefruit is a kick-ass fat-fighter. Researchers at the Scripps Clinic in La Jolla, California, have investigated its effect on weight loss and found that eating half a grapefruit before a meal can indeed help. The theory suggests that there is a physiological link between grapefruit and a reduction in insulin levels, which serves to impede fat storage. What's more, grapefruit contains cancer-fighting compounds such as liminoids and lycopene, and clocks in at only 39 calories per hemisphere.

Apples. The humble apple really is worth keeping about your person. Not only is it a portable, prepackaged powerhouse, loaded with vitamin C, fiber, sustaining sugars, and crunch, it is—if you shop wisely—likely to be a more local product than a banana, with all the health and environmental benefits that brings. Apples are also a superb source of pectin, a soluble fiber that can't be absorbed by the body but can be very handy on its way through. Pectin makes the apple a fiercely functional food: It is thought to limit the amount of fat your cells can absorb, it helps to balance blood-sugar levels, and it can even cause the stomach to empty more slowly, leaving you fuller longer. In addition to all this good stuff, pectin was recently found to have anticarcinogenic effects in the colon. There is also something aesthetically pleasing about an apple; its rounded heft in your hand, the roses on its cheeks, its ability to simultaneously explain the laws of gravity and dance with cloves in a pie. I'll give you six kiwis for a single Golden Delicious any day.

Olive oil. Scientists have recently discovered that oleic acid—a fatty acid found in abundance in olive oil, though also present in nuts and avocados—can trigger a reaction in the body that staves off hunger pangs. It is converted by the digestive system into a hormone called oleoylethanolamide: tricky to spell, yes, but a powerful no-diet dieting tool that will keep you satisfied between meals in a way that a bag of Skittles never could.

Flax seeds. A tiny, insubstantial sort of seed, true, but flax is a potent cocktail of edible goodies. Its scientific name, *Linum usitatissimum*, means "most useful"—and a brief saunter through its benefits proves why: Flax seeds have been shown to help control high blood pressure, promote bone health, lower cholesterol, and—important to us—boost the metabolism, which can help stimulate weight loss. These itsy seeds are rich in alpha-linolenic acid—that's an omega-3 fat—and they are a condensed source of antiviral, antioxidant lignans, together with all manner of vitamins and minerals, and, as a final parting shot, system-sweeping fiber. They taste vaguely nutty and are a superior addition to your morning cereal or oatmeal. Use the cold-pressed oil for salad dressings, but don't cook with it or you'll annihilate the goodness.

Lecithin. It might sound like a man-made nutraceutical (Can't you hear it? "Eat Less! Be Thin! With Lecithin™!"), but it is in fact a vital component of your body. Approximately one-third of the "dry weight" of your brain—I know, *eeew*, but bear with me here—is formed of the stuff. Lecithin is a fatlike substance produced in the liver, and it's essential for making each cell's protective membrane. That means it's responsible for the control of nutrients in and out, like a bouncer at a nightclub. It is high in B vitamins, particularly choline, which is blessed with the ability to break up fats. Beyond the science, all you really need to know is that lecithin is a good guy. You can find it in soybeans, eggs (the word itself is derived from the Greek word *likithos*, meaning egg yolk), grains, and brewer's yeast. It is your fat shield. Wear it well.

Garlic. In laboratory tests on rats, scientists at Israel's Weizmann Institute of Science found that garlic apparently prevents weight gain and, though the process is still only partially understood, may even lead to weight loss.[7] As far as I'm aware, they didn't test it as a vampire repellent—but really, I wouldn't be surprised if it could do that, too. Garlic is, says biochemist David Mirelman, a "wonder drug," brilliant at a whole range of jobs, from lowering blood pressure to treating diabetes—thanks to its active ingredient, allicin. It is this sulphurous compound that gives garlic its pungency, and, it is thought, protects cells and reduces fatty deposits. Even if you don't buy the hype, it's worth noting the hallowed place history reserves for garlic. It helped build the pyramids; it powered Greek athletes; it protected Roman centurions; Hippocrates himself recommended garlic for infections, wounds, leprosy, and digestive disorders. I recommend it for Pasta Puttanesca. Or bake it whole in its skin and spread it on bread.

Blueberries. In the pantheon of superfoods (small yawn), few are as comely and toothsome as the blueberry. These megaberries are powerfully antioxidant and rammed with sparkling vitamin C—which, as you'll recall from Step 11, is a vital tool for weight management.

Almonds. It's always worth remembering that the food industry is well-versed in promoting its products as wonder, super, über, and otherwise heroic. But, if you are to believe the hype, almonds are pretty much the food of the gods. Forget milk and honey—eat almonds. For years, scientists have been vaguely aware that people who regularly eat almonds tend to weigh less than people who don't. No one was entirely sure why or how—until a series of studies started to unveil the almond's secrets. One, from Purdue University, found that adding two servings of almonds to an existing diet had no effect on body weight or percentage of body fat per se, but it did satisfy hunger rather brilliantly. The researchers also found that the fiber in almonds seemed to block some of the fat they contain, keeping it from being digested and absorbed. To top it all off, preliminary research from an international group of universities suggests that eating almonds can reduce the impact that carb-rich food has on blood-sugar levels.[8] Too good to be true? Who knows? My feeling, in a nutshell, is give them a go. They're protein-packed, nutritious, and high in fiber. They don't smell, they don't leak, and they fit neatly (I have discovered) into the interior pocket of a Hermès Kelly bag.

Sunflower seeds. Packed with good fats. And iron. Zinc. Potassium, fiber, vitamins E and B$_1$, magnesium, selenium . . . enough already. The big sell is that they take *ages* to eat. A whole evening can be gone, and you've only consumed seven seeds, working, like a late-winter bird, for every last scrap. Genius.

36 THROW OUT THE FRYING PAN AND BUY A FIVE-LEVEL STEAMER

You'd fall off your chair if you knew how many calories you could save by simply going from fried to grilled and steamed. If you fancy fries, don't open a frosty bag and pour them into a deep-fat fryer; instead, chop up a potato and stick the wedges in a roasting pan with a bit of rosemary and a dash of olive oil. Rather than building an entire meal in a frying pan, build *up*, in a multistory steamer. Start on the ground floor with a delicate fillet of white fish, put some sugar snap peas in the next level up, and a handful of young spinach in the penthouse. Again, small changes, big calorie savings. Do some DIY and get building.

37 SURVIVE THE SNACK ATTACKS

I'm not a shrew. I know that you may need to keep your ghrelin in check with the occasional snack. Fine. But if you really must graze, do it mindfully and find a tasty low-cal treat that works for you. Rather than endless snacking on foods developed in laboratories and tested on rats, go natural. According to Hollywood lore, a good many A-listers rely on asparagus and parsley as snacks, because they believe these morsels repress hunger and reduce bloating. (Actually, they don't work, though they are mildly diuretic and may make you feel momentarily lighter.) Follow this advice, instead.

Be prepared. Don't leave the house hungry, or you will walk blindly toward the nearest donut shop. Keep an apple in your handbag (see Step 35 to know why). My great friend Valerie always carries a boiled egg in her handbag, but then she is a trifle odd.

Wow your mouth with the occasional taste treat. It's your mouth, so you decide what that treat is. At the moment (and you may well find them disagreeable), I'm going with Fisherman's Friend Cherry Menthols—a small bomb of curiously punchy flavor contained in a humble 3-calorie lozenge. You can find something similar near the checkout line at your local pharmacy. You might prefer an orange Tic Tac. Or that chewing gum that's so full of menthol flavor that it makes your eyes water and your hair stand on end. Whatever it is, the idea is to flirt with your mouth from time to time—giving it powerful hits of taste—so that it doesn't lead you into temptation. Better an Altoid than three rounds of Nutella on toast.

Look for leaves. You don't need a PhD in nutrition to work this one out, but do try to snack on things that *grow*—olives, blueberries, pickles, baby beets, seeds of any and all descriptions, plum tomatoes, cucumber sticks, baby carrots. Keep them close. Dip them in hummus or tzatziki, if you have to. In a pretty little bowl, right here in front of my keyboard, I have cherry tomatoes on the vine. (Their fragrance reminds me of the intense tang of my grandmother's greenhouse in high summer, the air thick with heat and the buzz of insects, the tomato plants giving off their provocative green perfume.) I also have a handful of fat pink radishes—those long ones that look like they're blushing—and some bright-white cauliflower florets cold from the fridge. I know it's not a Twix bar, but it does fill that snacky time of day you get to when you're working, when your jaw is bored and your stomach is not exactly demanding lunch, but just suggesting that it would like a little something.

Eat heat. Avoid bland stuff, and snack instead on fiery pickles, hot chiles, and strong flavors that your brain will remember. (I'm into piquillo peppers at the moment. Grown in northern Spain, these babies are hand-picked, roasted over an open fire, peeled, and packed in their own juices in a jar.) You might prefer Manzanilla olives stuffed with a salty kick of anchovy, sweet pickled guindilla chiles, or skinny slivers of spicy chorizo. As you nibble on these passionate snacks, amuse yourself with the news that researchers at Laval University in Canada have recently found that eating hot peppers can speed up your metabolism, cool your cravings, and lower your calorie intake. Apparently capsaicin—a compound found in jalapeño and cayenne peppers—"temporarily stimulates your body to release more stress hormones, which speeds up your metabolism and causes you to burn more calories." Ginger and black pepper are thought to have similar thermogenic effects, according to research at Maastricht University.[9] So fire 'em up!

As a last resort . . . If you must, have a Snackwell. Though they contain sugar and, of course, calories, they are fat-free. They are still 50 calories each, though, so don't get to the last crumb of one and immediately embark on another. You will, however, have just enjoyed an illusion of fat, housed in a whole heap of taste. Otherwise, go for . . .

Home-popped popcorn. Madonna's snack of choice feels equally decadent but is low in those devilish calories (so long as you don't slather it with butter, cheese topping, or a combination of the two).

38 IF YOU'RE FEELING PECKISH, BRUSH YOUR TEETH

Works every time. Some folks—including Matthew McConaughey, apparently—believe that a new taste in the mouth sends a signal to the brain that you are full, and brushing accomplishes this without any calories at all. It will also please your dentist.

39 ORDER ONE DESSERT, TWO FORKS

Twice the fun, half the calories. There are countless other clever ways to eat, of course.

* Order two appetizers and no main.

* Take a vow of dessert abstinence, with amnesty every third Tuesday.

* Choose labor-intensive food—lobster or crab, perhaps—that will occupy your hands and mouth. Foods like this are fantastically sociable and they suck up great amounts of time.

* Similarly, crispy Peking Duck in a Chinese restaurant is time-consuming and pleasing, engaging both conversation and the effort of many fingers.

* Ditto artichokes: so sociable. Dip the leaves in vinaigrette, rather than melted butter.

* Choose edamame (soy beans) from a sushi bar, or indeed from a little ceramic bowl planted on your desk (just 3 grams of fat per 100 grams!).

* Satay, it should be noted, is a sociable food that's less appealing on several counts. It's usually fried, it comes with a heavy peanut sauce, and there is always the prospect that you will do as I once did in a very upscale restaurant: While attempting to pry a chicken chunk from its stick, I applied a bit too much force and a missile of meat flew across the room like a superhero and landed in the handbag of a fellow diner two tables away. She didn't notice. I didn't tell her. It feels so good to confess.

40 DON'T BE A TRASHIONISTA

I'm the first to adhere to the anonymous adage that "there are four basic food groups: milk chocolate, dark chocolate, white chocolate, and chocolate truffles." We all know that there are times in a life, and times of the month, when a little cocoa can go a long way toward making you feel loved and human and personable again. No one is asking you to endure a Decaflon (according to the *Washington Post*, this is "the grueling event of getting through the day consuming only things that are good for you"). And don't straitjacket yourself with the cardiologist's diet ("if it tastes good, spit it out"). A life of deprivation is, after all, no life at all—and what we're after here, remember, is sustainable, permanent, attainable change.

Fine. But, when you *do* treat yourself, try a little bit of lovely, not a whole lot of junk. Make it a fantastic oozy Brie, not cheese on toast; a bottle of the good stuff, not a splash of something from a box; a couple of squares of dark Godiva chocolate—not, not, not a family-size

Hershey's bar. And make sure that occasional treats stay occasional. Otherwise, like Hansel and Gretel, you will be following a trail of tasty morsels all the way back to the old, fat you.

If you are going to have a periodic off-script splurge, you may as well go for things that have other benefits. For example:

* **Red wine.** Though relatively high in calories, the odd glass of vino rosso is also high in resveratrol, thought to boast a host of benefits—not least that it may offset the negative effects of gluttony. Studies at Maastricht University in the Netherlands suggest that grape seed extract can reduce calorie intake; meanwhile, researchers at Harvard Medical School also found that resveratrol slows down the aging process in nonmammalian animals.[10] Doesn't necessarily mean it will work for you and me, but let's give it a try, shall we?

* **Butter.** Contains conjugated linoleic acid, which is thought to help fight breast cancer. What a bonus. Even so, keep it as a treat, not a habit. Use olive oil or rapeseed oil for cooking, and have a little bit of butter sometimes. On Sunday, say, with hot toast and a good cup of coffee.

* **Proper chocolate.** New research says that cocoa may well contain more antioxidants than green tea does. And, as every marketing executive knows, it is thought to have aphrodisiac and serotonin-boosting properties, which can certainly get a girl through a miserable Monday in one piece. As Gwyneth Paltrow confessed to *Grazia* magazine: "Once in a while I'll have some chocolate cake." The operative words in this sentence are "once in a while"—*not* "chocolate" and "cake." Remember that all chocolate contains fat and sugar, but some chocolates are fatter and sweeter than others. Always go for the top-drawer stuff. Perhaps something from Godiva or Ghirardelli. Either way, next time you bite into a truffle or a dark chocolate turtle, don't think "Damn calories!" Think "Mmm, antioxidant flavonoids."

And if you do occasionally fall off the wagon, treat it as a momentary hiccup, not a Greek tragedy. Move on. There are better things to do than mope. Like? Well, like reading the next chapter, for one.

5

HOW TO DRESS THIN . . .

AND CHEAT THE WORLD

You've come a long way, baby. You've discovered ways to trim and pare, ways to think thin and eat smart. Now for the divinely easy part. You only want to diet because you think you look fat, right? So don't look fat! What you need is the fashion editor's inside scoop on diet dressing— all of those cunning, stunning little tricks that get your wardrobe to do the work, so you don't have to.

41 GET A DIET DRESS

As Mark Twain so neatly noted, "Clothes make the man. Naked people have little or no influence in society." Dead right, but what he failed to add is that when it comes to the *woman*, clothes don't just make her: They can also break her. It all hinges on the dozens of tiny questions and decisions that flit through your barely conscious mind as you gaze into your closet in the morning. Should you risk wearing your old jeans to take the kids to school? (Probably not.) Is a tube top acceptable for a meeting with your real estate agent? (Possibly, but only if you'd like him to show you a certain type of property.) Can you take your cleavage to church? (Yes, but make it wear a scarf.)

Getting it wrong is a constant threat—a problem that barely afflicts men, who know that a suit, by and large, will get them through any scenario without unduly troubling the eye. But women need clothes we can trust, clothes we can rely on in a storm or a heat wave, clothes that will take us gently by the hand and lead us through thick and thin and all manner of tribulations in between. And most of all, most of us, most of the time, need a Diet Dress.

This fabled garment is the absolute axis of a slim life, and though its specifics are wholly personal, there are a handful of rules that apply to us all. A Diet Dress is almost all in the cut, which is why it's worth spending both time and money on its purchase. There are designers who, having studied the arc and arch of the female form, are experts at cutting a Diet Dress. By way of example, Alber Elbaz, designer at Lanvin, cuts a superlative sleeveless dress that somehow manages to conceal the ugly underarm wobble we all despise. Perhaps you love your arms, but hate your sloping shoulders? In that case, look for a little padding in the area to give you a lift. You might want to rediscover your waist or entertain the idea of a bracelet sleeve, the better to show off an elegant wrist. It doesn't really matter what it is: The point is, you and you alone must find your asset and invest in it.

Though it works admirably hard, clocking up hour after hour on duty, the Diet Dress should be an unobtrusive element in your wardrobe—not the wicked, foxy number that introduces itself to strangers at parties. Not the one that everybody will notice and remember the next time you wear it. Not the one that makes you think about it every third minute, like a newborn infant, demanding your attention because it has risen up your thigh or dipped down to reveal your bra strap. No. A Diet Dress is the strong and silent type. Reliable. Quietly confident.

Its shape will depend, largely, on yours. My own Diet Dress is in a delicious midnight blue silk jersey, the color of deep water. It is high at the neck—a surprise to me, that—with an asymmetric hem, bell sleeves, and a dropped waist. If this sounds hideous, well, hands off, it's mine. The point is that this particular dress makes *me* feel fabulous. And, perhaps more to the point, it makes me feel thin. It is lengthy and languid, elongating rather than widening my body. It clings in all the right places and tactfully skims over the wrong ones, and it is my Diet Dress chiefly because of the body that inhabits it. Your Diet Dress will probably be another species entirely. It may feature something sturdy in the bodice or have a full skirt to camouflage heavy thighs. It may reveal your fabulous décolleté or thrill bystanders with a glimpse of your knees. It may dance over your chest, only to make a big play of your delightful waist. Only you will recognize when you have found your glory dress—you'll know from your smile as you introduce it to the mirror for the first time.

Discovering the cut that best suits your body requires both perseverance and ingenuity. Once you find it, clasp it to your grateful bosom and never let it go. Here are a few hints to get you going.

* **An A-line is a kind line.** This shape manages the diplomatic trick of making your shoulders appear less broad, while skating over the usual off-limits areas of belly, butt, and thighs. (BBT—that classic sandwich of little-loved body bits.) It's what fashion writers are wont to call a "no-brainer" dress, because it marries form to function and you needn't give it a bit of thought.

* **Shall I wrap that for you, madam?** If you possess a substantial chest, this one's for you, as it escorts the eye down the inviting gulley of its plunge to arrive at a waist made all the more petite because of the structure above and the rippling skirt below. The seminal wrap, of course, came from Diane von Furstenberg, way back in the seventies, when it ruled at Studio 54, doing disco and generally causing a wicked stir. By the middle of that decade, von Furstenberg was turning out 15,000 dresses a week. As she says: "The wrap dress made women feel what they wanted to feel like . . . free and sexy. . . . It also fitted in with the sexual revolution: A woman who chose to could be out of it in less than a minute!" It was liberating for women, and—vitally—it was also unexpectedly forgiving. "What is so special about it," von Furstenberg says of the dress she reintroduced in 1997, "is that it's a very traditional form of clothing. It's like a toga, it's like a kimono, without buttons, without a zipper. What made my wrap dresses different is that they were made out of jersey and they sculpted the body." Aha! Sculpted. That's the key—and until you've given one a spin, you won't truly understand its benevolent blessings, the way it fires up a figure, ignores a bulge, and is uncommonly kind to a waist when your pants feel that bit too tight. "I would say the wrap dress is better when you are a bit curvier," says its inventor. Go buy one—now!

* **The empire, on which the sun never sets.** If, like me, you have a demanding tummy, then the empire line will love you. It's obvious why—that just-below-the-breast seam allows any kind of malarkey to be hidden by the looser fabric below. Breathe easy. Diet Dress to the rescue.

* **Drop your waist, drop a dress size.** If you are thick in the middle—and darlings, we know who we are—then the simple expedient of a dropped waist will achieve much the same effect as an empire line, tricking the eye away from your belly—in this case, allowing attention to rest, comfortably, on your hip. The hip is a mighty fine place to rest, as women who adore low-rise jeans well testify: The body is stretched, the bottom shrinks, and the woman inside shines like a sunbeam and rocks the room.

* **When in doubt, get Lucky (or Galaxy, or Power).** There's usually a dress of the season, and by some genius law of fashion physics, it is generally a Diet Dress. Thus, Roland Mouret's Galaxy dress a while back was an absolute master class in the art. It held you in, pushed you up, and managed that trick of turning something loose and soft (your BBT) into something altogether more taut and tantalizing. It did

WHY A DRESS?

There's always a "piece" that distills a season, a garment that will whisk you from last month to next month in the mere wink of an eye. If you inhabit the right sort of places, you might occasionally find fashion folk in huddles, saying things like "It's all about the cardigan!" or "Pants! We're going big on pants!" This season, it may be tulip skirts, next it could be pedal pushers or peacoats. But usually, usually it's a dress, the undisputed stalwart of style. The reason for its towering popularity lies in its versatility, dress-up-ability, femininity, and—crucially—the fact that you chuck it over your head and you're done. As designer Alber Elbaz of Lanvin puts it, "What I love about the dress isn't just the prettiness and romance, but also the simplicity. I love the zip-in and zip-out. It's the most modern uniform."

this by the mere expedience of its cut: its figure-framing capped sleeves, its sinuous zip from nape to hem, its darted, engineered fabric carved to flick and furl about the body like a shower of kisses. More recently, you may have noticed the Lucky dress from Issa's designer Daniella Helayel, as seen on Scarlett Johansson, Hilary Swank, and Kristin Davis. The fashion world is unanimous: This is a high-performance dress virtually guaranteed to make you feel brilliant. How? "I think the Lucky is such a hit because it flatters every body shape," says Helayel. "I started designing dresses because I couldn't find any that suited my own body—I'm Brazilian and curvy. It just seems to be one of those dresses that everyone feels good in." The square neckline flatters most busts, the stitched bodice is a torso-tamer, the full skirt gives the welcome impression of slim legs, slim waist, slim you (while coasting considerably over your butt). Alternatively, the Preen Power Dress—a regular in the label's collections—will do something similar with a bit more slice and a lot more va-va-voom. "We set out for it to be the ultimate cocktail dress that pulls you in and gives you body confidence," says Preen designer Justin Thornton. The illusion is achieved in several cunning ways: Wide straps slim the shoulder (and, crucially, allow you to wear a bra); tucks and pleats of high-tensile Elastane swerve around the body, pumping up assets and navigating trouble spots; the tube skirt, which pulls everything in like a dog herding sheep, is softened by a second tier, so you don't look like a waitress in a girly bar; and the whole thing is lined with a second skin of "Powernet," a tough contouring mesh used in corsets. Holy smoke.

42 FIND THE RIGHT JEANS

I seem to be surrounded by perfect bottoms. Everywhere I turn, there's another one—getting into a cab, easing itself onto a bar stool, running up that hill. Over the years, I have become something of an expert in the derriere department, like one of those construction workers who can rate a passing woman's bottom on a scale of 1 to 10, even while troweling mortar onto bricks and eating a Big Mac.

I take great interest in other girls' bottoms in the same way that I'm fascinated by their kitchens (if they're fabulous) and their relationships (if they're not). It's a hobby founded on envy, of course, but finessed by the thought that, with a little effort and a lot of abstinence, I too could have a bottom that behaves impeccably in a bikini.

The best behind I know of personally belongs to my friend Freya, and it is always housed in a pair of red-hot jeans. Hot jeans have the right label (True Religion, Sass & Bide, Citizens of Humanity, Hudson, J Brand), in the same way that substandard jeans don't. But here's the thing: It was only when I went on vacation with Freya and her super-bum that I realized that it was *all* in the jeans. Her bottom was pretty average when let loose, so to speak. It was those jeans that made hers a butt worth watching.

Yup, nothing on earth can cup and cradle your assets so effectively as the perfect pair of jeans. "They are," says fashion designer Mary Quant, "the greatest invention ever. . . ." But the question is, how do you get your hands on that elusive beast, the perfect pair? As with most matters of style, it depends a lot on what you've got; a pear cannot hope to be a peach using jean therapy alone. But you can maximize your assets. Here's how.

* Try, try, try. Then, when you find perfection, buy, buy, buy.
* Generally speaking, big bottoms look smaller in a boy-cut jean—invariably, they'll have a shorter rise (the distance between crotch and waistband), which minimizes the area covered. Hipsters create a similar optical illusion.
* Denim has immense tummy-flattening capabilities. Says fashion designer Katharine Hamnett, "There's an element of corsetry in jeans cutting—[denim is] tough enough to hold you in." A flat-lying waistband sitting just below the navel is generally the most flattering—though it depends entirely on the contours of your body. If you need to tame a tummy, a higher waist will keep everything in line, restrained by all that glorious, dependable denim. Wear a longer top if you need to, to mask the magic.
* Women's jeans are traditionally tapered below the knee and roomier at the thigh, which tends to shorten and add bulk to a figure. Instead, choose a straight-leg jean, though I strongly support resurrecting the trend for boot-cut jeans, the most flattering fashion ever bestowed upon womankind, with their implicit guarantee to elongate the leg and shrink the bottom. What more, really, could you ask of a pair of jeans? Keep them lean at the thigh, with a sharp flare from knee to hem.
* Buy a size that sits comfortably rather than one that clings to your thighs like a child on his first day at school.
* Buy them long and wear heels. Adding height is, of course, the most obvious way to look leggy when you're not. To diminish the tarty overtone, wear a heeled boot. And only original stitching looks acceptable at your hem, so buy one pair of jeans for flats and another for heels.
* If you have thighs of a certain size—I'm not pointing, I'm just saying—

beware of jeans with those jazzy bleached or distressed zones on the legs that simply draw attention to the blights in your life.

* If you're 17 and built like a sapling, go for bleached. Otherwise, buy a classic dark blue; it is most forgiving.

* Whatever you buy, pay close attention to the back pockets, which will alter the dimensions of a bottom by leading the eye in a certain direction: Levi's masterstroke on its timeless 501s was to add stitching in a V-shape, giving the illusion of a smaller, neater rump . . . surely every girl's dearest, deepest wish?

* If you have a Houdini belly (one that's forever trying to escape), take a look at Tummy Tuck Jeans from Not Your Daughter's Jeans. They feature a high Lycra content and a patented crisscross panel designed to firm you up. Go to notyourdaughtersjeans.com to find a store where you can test-drive a pair.

* Once you've bagged your dream jeans, wear them often. Wear them as a statement of style, not as a bored basic. Better still, wear your skinniest, tightest pair, particularly if you're feeling fat. (Do this at home if you can't face the public.) Trust me: Nothing will do more to keep you away from that leftover piece of pie.

43 CHOOSE FIT CLOTHES, NOT FAT CLOTHES

Never wear a shapeless sweater in the hope that it will hide a multitude of sins; it won't. What you need are properly fitted clothes, tight to the torso, fitted to your figure. This is the most flattering and slimming silhouette for any body shape, and you will benefit from it in an instant. If you can afford to, ditch your budget habit (cheap often means clunky) and invest in fewer, more-tailored, more-expensive clothes. Don't be afraid to have garments altered to your specifications and measurements—not too tight, but just right—even if you bought them off the rack in a chain store. Tailored garments will shave off pounds, not ounces. Rather brilliantly, tailoring is one of the few fashion concepts that looks better as you age. It won't give you the time of day until you're 33, and then it's all over you like an expensive suit. It is simply one of those good things that comes to those who wait—and, as many a former model will tell you, a great tailor will do *far* more for you than a great surgeon will.

If in doubt (and not yet in debt), my strong advice is to reach for couturier Antony Price. The man who dressed Roxy Music, Duran Duran, Princess Diana, and every glittery Glamazon in between, is known, in certain circles, as "the doctor." His forte, based on decades of finessing and refinement, is illusion. "I'm the man who has spent 40 years measuring and studying women's bodies," Price says. "Not just thin women. Everyday real women. Real bosoms. Real problems. Women who have no [boobs] and want them, and women who want them smaller. I *build* frocks."

The bottom line, he says, is that "shapely women look better in fitted clothes. If you have material hanging, you just look like a salad bowl with drooping lettuce. Corsetry enables you to take the fabric of the dress and bang it right against your skin where you immediately lose a size or two. Smooth, no bits or lumps." Just what the doctor ordered, right?

44 UNDERSTAND THE POWER OF PERFECT BLACK PANTS

Work tirelessly until you discover a pair that flatters you. Then buy three pairs. Keep them pristine, dry-cleaned, and pressed, not in a jumbled heap on the floor. Why? Because they are the most forgiving, the most friendly, the most fantastic garment ever to walk the face of the earth. Now, I know they don't seem like much, hanging there on the rack, minding their own business. I can almost feel your disappointment. But bear with me. Black pants are my "desert island" garment. They can save the hour, the day, the outfit. They can take you to work and then escort you to the movies, then on to cocktails, dinner, and home to collapse in front of the TV. They'll get along with anything—a T-shirt, a tux, a tissue-silk top scattered with seed pearls and silver sequins; they'll meet any color head on and make it look good. They're versatile and vivacious, comfortable and cool. They're the sartorial equivalent of that lovely boyfriend your mom liked but you thought was too safe—and, like with him, you'll never know what you had till they're gone. Safe, perhaps. But my word, they're handsome.

Make sure, then, that they're not overly trendy. I have one fabulous pair that are wide-legged, high-waisted, with cuffs and a whole heap of swaggering attitude. Fine for days when you want people to say, "Wow, check out those pants!" But the perfect pair simply needs to keep quiet and get on with the job at hand. Go for a simple straight leg and a fit that suits the quirks of your own figure. This means—yes—you need to try and try again. I find a flat-front with a knife-edge crease works best for me, but you may prefer a boot-cut or a low waist. You will also need to think weight—not yours, but theirs. Have several pairs to cover all eventualities and weather conditions. I suggest you procure each of the following, just to cover your bases.

* **Black wool suit pants.** Not synthetic, not a heavy weight, not ones that look like they're trying too hard. What you want is the kind of pants you barely know are there, like the quiet kid at school who goes on to win the Nobel Prize for physics.

* **Black denim jeans.** Workaday stuff, sure, but immune to stains and

TO CUT A LONG STORY SHORT . . .

The hem of your pants ought to hit ½ inch from the ground, comfortably on the top arch of your foot. Unless your desert island pants are designed to be worn cropped or trailing the floor like a lovelorn Ophelia, then make sure the hem stops right there, having pulled off the twin tricks of making your legs look long and your feet look petite.

scuffs, and therefore a wardrobe winner every time. Will work hard on your behalf, covering both day and night shifts, back-to-back if necessary.

* **Black cotton capris.** Wear with an embroidered top or a loose linen shirt, and you've got "summer in the city" down pat.

* **Black velvet jeans.** A garment that will party till dawn and then get up and take the kids to school.

* **Black satin pants.** Just so chic.

45 BE PARTICULAR ABOUT WHERE YOU BUY YOUR CLOTHES: SIZES DIFFER, AND CERTAIN DESIGNERS WILL FLATTER YOUR BODY BEST

Getting dressed in the 21st century is, as we all know, a pretty haphazard affair, but it is made all the more complicated by our increasingly unruly bodies and the apparent reluctance of the design world to take the tiniest bit of notice. While manufacturers insist on making clothes to fit the traditional hourglass shape, only 8 percent of women are built that way anymore, according to a recent report from North Carolina State University.[1] It's a bit like car manufacturers refusing to make anything but car-seat covers for fifties Corvettes: Much of what's on the market simply doesn't fit.

Designer Katharine Hamnett—never one to toe the party line in fashion—has long been mightily aggravated by the issue. "The fashion industry ignores the true size of women at its peril," she warns. "As to why they do, stupidity is the only reason I can think of. It is the result of adhering unthinkingly to a tradition."

Daisy Lowe, model and muse, seems to have given the issue some thought and has arrived at her own conclusion: "I love curvaceousness," she says. "Curvy girls are the sexiest girls. If clothes were built for curvier women, which is most of the population, one: people would look better; two: designers would sell more clothes, and three: they wouldn't have to use tiny anorexic models. . . ."

WHY APPLES AND PEARS ARE BANANAS

For some reason, it is currently fashionable to size up a body, judge it, label it—and then dress it according to a template, as if commanded by Moses himself. All over the country, and perhaps the world, it's Apples or Pears. As a fashion columnist for a Sunday newspaper in the United Kingdom, I regularly hear from women trying in vain to ascertain their shape, as if labeling a body will somehow make it look better in a halter-neck dress. "Am I a Spoon?" comes a plaintive e-mail from Wolverhampton; "I think I'm a Flower Pot," writes Rita in Devon. "Is this normal?" No, Rita, it's not. It is ludicrous.

Pigeonholing our blameless bodies in this way somehow misses the point of getting dressed at all. Fashion, if you're living it and loving it, is an intimate and glorious thing. It thrives on personality and attitude, character and lifestyle; it is sparked by age, contained by budget, driven by dreams, and influenced by a whole lot of other things that have nothing to do with the size of your bottom in relation to the width of your hips. What works for one size 14 won't necessarily work for another; what looks delicious on one "Spoon" will make another look like a Ladle. If style truly worked in this plodding, reductive way, we'd all dress like drones—neutered, neutralized, and desperately dull at parties.

You are not an abstract shape, hanging there in the ether, tethered by neither temperament nor taste. You are a person, and the most effective way of dressing depends largely on what makes you feel good. To ascertain your shape, then, don't look in a book. Let your clothing be your guide: Your favorite jeans will tell you so much more than your scale—or those Apples and Pears—ever could.

True enough. But until the fashion industry shakes itself from its stupor, the best way to find labels that love your shape is to clear a morning and book a session with a fashion adviser or personal shopper. There are undiscovered labels out there that will work for you, and a professional will be able to ferret them out before you can say "Does that come in chartreuse?" They know very well that clothes don't come in standard sizes and that one shop's 12 is another's 14. They understand the quirks of cut and fit that are unique to a particular label. There is great value in a little expert advice, just so long as you keep your eyes open and your plastic under strict control. So why let the A-list hog all the personal services? Go grab a bit for yourself. Google "personal shopper" and your city name, and see if you can find some local help. Or, if you have a Macy's or Saks nearby, make an appointment to meet with one of their personal shoppers.

One final note: I recommend that you wear your good undies and have a bikini-line appointment before you embark on a dressing room encounter with your new best friend. You'll be glad you did.

46 BEWARE OF—AND STOP KIDDING YOURSELF ABOUT—VANITY SIZING

It is possible that, many moons ago, the world's clothing manufacturers got together for a PowerPoint presentation called "How to Keep Your Customer Satisfied." And right there at the top of the list, in big neon capital letters, was this simple directive:

LIE.

Stick a smaller size on bigger pants! It really is so easy and so very appealing. Yes, but it's a honey trap, people, and you don't have to be a complete ditz to fall for it. Here's a little fairy tale to illustrate my point: One day, not so long ago, I discovered from the interior of a pair of jeans that I was a size 8. A size 8! That's a 4 in the States! As you might expect, I was thrilled to tiny little pieces and bought two pairs before the shop assistant could draw breath. I had size-8 friends, of course— more associates, really—women who looked so fabulous in shorts that you'd want to take yourself outside and jump off the curb and into the path of an oncoming ice cream truck. But now, here I was, a size 8! I would spread the good news, I'd yell it from the rooftops, there'd be rejoicing in the . . . hang on a second. These jeans were suspiciously roomy. I got them home, and found that they bore precisely the same dimensions as the old size 10s that I'd shoved to the back of my closet. I'd been tricked.

"Vanity sizing is all about making women feel thinner than they are," says Yasmin Sewell, fashion director at a small London boutique. As she told the *Times*, "We want to wear brands that flatter us. We also work with several celebrity stylists who practice vanity sizing to keep their A-list clients happy. They will cut out a size 14 label and sew in a size 10 label. It's the same thing."

Now, I don't give two hoots what size you happen to be, but the issue is that these vanity sizes bear no relation to how much space we actually take up in a bus or a bathtub. And the truth is—brace yourselves—that women have been growing dramatically wider and heavier since the fifties, while the sizing we see on our labels has simply grown to accommodate our new girth. According to SizeUSA, between 1941 and 2004, American women added an average of 7 inches around the waist. The average Caucasian American woman between the ages of 36 and 45 now measures 41-34-43. Black women in that age group average 43-37-46. We may smirk to ourselves, as we climb into a size-8 skirt, that Marilyn Monroe was a size 14. Hah! we think, breathing in to get that zipper up, what a monumental fatty she was! Marilyn, for the record, had a 22-inch waist. In today's parlance, that makes her a pretty small size 8.

Vanity sizing is now so widespread that a peculiar vacuum has emerged at the lower end of the spectrum as smaller sizes are commandeered for larger clothes, giving rise to the 0 and 00 that have caused so much excitement lately. Any time now, we'll be into negative numbers, worn by women who are the shape and size of julienned vegetables. "I'm a minus 4!" they'll chirp from behind the changing-room curtain. "By the laws of mathematics, I no longer exist!"

The psychology behind the practice is enough to make you rue the day you were born a woman. Apparently, 10 percent of us cut the tags out of our clothes so we don't have to see the size on a daily basis. The rest of us prefer to live the lie, abetted by those cunning manufacturers who know that the smaller the size, the better we feel—ergo, the more we'll buy.

What this means for women of any size is that you can't trust a label, you *must* try your clothes on. At L.L.Bean, for instance, a size 10 is significantly larger than a size 10 at Abercrombie and Fitch, with its younger clientele. French Connection's 10s are notoriously minuscule, and sometimes there's a more insidious reason for that. Brix Smith-Start, of London designer-boutique Start, tells the *Times*, with admirable candor, that sometimes designers size their clothes that way "because they want to keep big people out of them. Having fat people wear your clothes is not good for a brand's image. It's a fact of life," she says.

True enough. The brute fact is that certain design houses simply don't want heavier people wearing their collections—perhaps because beautiful, slimline people perpetuate the myth that only beautiful, slimline people wear their clothes. With many top-end labels, as Smith-Start says, "if you are curvy . . . forget it."

Clearly, different design houses and manufacturers have wildly opposing views of what makes a size 10, 14, or 18. I was once (briefly, years ago) the in-house model for the fashion designer Nicole Farhi, and they used my funny, silly body as the template for a size 10 just because I happened to be hanging around doing the filing. It's as random as that.

STICK IT TO THE SIZEISTS

What to do about the boutiques that refuse to stock anything above a size 8? The designers who produce clothes only fit for mannequins? Boycott their handbags, people! Shame them by complaining loudly at the register. Write letters to the *New York Times*. Picket! I'm not expecting all labels to accommodate all sizes, but more availability for those of us who fall within the bell curve of normal would be smashing, thanks ever so much.

Little wonder that a 2003 survey found that 50 percent of consumers say they have difficulty finding clothes that fit well.[2] And you need clothes that *fit*, rather than flatter to deceive, regardless of that pesky little number breathing down your neck and whispering velvet compliments in your ear. Shove yourself into clothes that are the wrong size and you'll very likely look fat. Or stupid. Possibly both. Ignore the numbers and concentrate on the look. That, after all, is what matters most.

17 FIND *YOUR* SHOP

As Alexandra Shulman, editor of British *Vogue*, once told me, "It helps to know the designers that suit you, to find your shop, so you're not starting from scratch every time. . . . Having some idea of your own style, your strengths and weaknesses, helps—although, of course, they do change as you get older. Personally, I find it much harder to get away with boho dressing than I once did. You can so easily look like an aging [psychic]."

Indeed. In my experience, one productive visit to a beloved shop is worth a dozen schizophrenic trips along Main Street in a desperate search for the New You. Leave that to Madonna's stylists, and concentrate instead on a confidence-building, I-Am-Who-I-Am approach to shopping. Why do you think Kate Moss always wears J Brand jeans? Why does Angelina Jolie swear by her Anya Hindmarch bags? Not because these women don't have all the choice in the world, but because they have *made* a choice: They've found a faithful fashion friend and they're not about to change allegiance just because the wind has changed direction.

Once you have found the place that works for you—it may be a certain boutique, a particular designer, a chain store that feels like home—stick with it. Not religiously, but regularly. Don't be too promiscuous. Personally, I have been so hooked on Gap for the past decade that I get a bit antsy if I haven't rifled through the racks in a few weeks. It works for me. It may not work for you. Once you have discovered your shop, keep it close, keep it constant; use it as a cornerstone of your look. Then throw curveballs at it to pep things up.

48 BUY THE RIGHT SWIMSUIT

Every year, it happens. You look up from Easter and what do you know? Bikini time again. The most challenging weeks of your life are looming on the sun-kissed horizon, and you've just spent the last 2 weeks waist-deep in Cadbury eggs. In your mind's eye, you're Bo Derek emerging from the surf. You're Halle Berry in *Die Another Day!* You're Brigitte Bardot at Club 55! In reality, you're deluded, and you need all the help you can get, and fast. So, to all ye about to set sail for the shops to find that rare treasure, the bikini that, through the magic of a Lycra-rich waistband, will turn you into Scarlett Johansson, well, here's the skinny, my friends.

* There are classics in this game, and no one should leave home during a hot spell without the reliable armor of a well-cut black one-piece. Stifle those yawns. Like the little black dress, this is the very backbone of a successful wardrobe, and without it, you'll merely wobble along on the very periphery of beach chic. If black feels dull, turn to your accessories to make the splash you want: a giant bag in a floral print, a pair of spangled flip-flops, even big wooden beads (not to be worn as you dive into the deep end, or you'll knock yourself out).

* If you want your bikini to *work*, rather than simply take it easy on a lounger, you need to look for the following:

   1. Underwiring, which will stop your breasts from heading down Mexico way.

   2. A top with clip fastenings, not ties: These will give you added stability and eliminate the exhausted-looking flop of so many bad bikini tops.

   3. A tie-side bottom. Paradoxically, these are forgiving and won't bite into your rump like a wide-side can.

   4. High-leg bottoms to elongate a leg. (But be aware that these also demand exhibition-class depilation.)

   5. Confidence. This means that, when entering the water, you try not to fiddle with your bikini. You look fine, really. Pulling fabric from between your cheeks won't improve matters one iota and may serve to make things worse.

* Better yet, buy a Miraclesuit. Having spent most of my life—or at least the beach-bound portion of it—wearing smart little bikinis in Aegean blue, I recently discovered that I need a little helping hand if I am to look even the same *species* as a Penelope Cruz or a Helen Mirren (a woman 20 years my senior who makes me want to bay at the moon in jealous anguish). Still, as Helen herself knows, at a certain age, we all require a push here, a pick-up there. A bit of illusion. And this, dear reader, is where the Miraclesuit comes in. Tag line: "Look 10 pounds lighter in 10 seconds." Way to go! The cut has a hint of the fifties about it, with a substantial bottom, an elegant neckline, and a tremendous capacity to contain, thanks to a fabric with several times the tensile strength of Lycra. As a result, they make you walk like a screen goddess and look like a babe. Dynamite. All this comes at a cost. (Most are in the $125 to $150 range, though less-expensive versions are increasingly available.) There's also the vaguely unsettling sense that you've waltzed back in time to an era when women were tied to the stove and bound by their formidable underwear. Still, what price wouldn't we pay to look good on the beach?

* Of course, you could always rest easy in the comforting embrace of a beach caftan. It may not be the very pinnacle of cool, but there's no shame in it. This is easily one of the best fashion inventions of recent times, marrying as it does a nonchalant ethnicity with an unfussy chic. More to the point, it covers an entire catechism of sins and allows the wearer to feel, just for this short time, that they live on the same planet as Elizabeth Hurley. Bliss—not to mention a bonus for anyone who happens to be sitting behind you as you dive for the Frisbee on the soft white sand.

49 RECOGNIZE THAT THERE ARE SOME CLOTHES YOU SHOULD NEVER WEAR

Leafing through the *New York Times* recently, I came across this pearl of sartorial wisdom: "A leather belt works well over knits." Oh really? Have you tried it? In the interest of research (I put in the hours for you, really

I do), I buckled a wide leather belt at waist level over my old fisherman's sweater—and what did I look like? A roll of fiberglass insulation. Bottom line: A leather belt *never* works well over knits, unless you are built like a broom handle, and even then your friends will very likely discuss how dumpy you've become behind your back.

This got me thinking. While I have always been scrupulous with the truth when ruminating upon the complexities of fashion, I am suspicious that my contemporaries out there are sometimes less than entirely honest. To put things straight, I have compiled the following checklist of Style Lies that you may want to cut out and keep, perhaps in your purse, to be pulled out when confronted with a pile of duplicitous glossy magazines at the hairdressers.

1. It is not okay to wear a miniskirt past the age of 39. I am 40. Trust me. There is a cut-off point, and this is it.

2. Unless you are a MacDonald or a Campbell or a model for Burberry, plaid is not the answer to winter dressing.

3. Bags shaped like "things" (toy dogs, flowerpots, threatened wildlife) are not clever. They are idiotic. If you want to carry around a small animal, get a Chihuahua.

4. Ochre is not an "It Color." Along with a host of other shades, it is very tough to wear, whatever Giorgio Armani would have us believe. I include on my list tangerine (and, while we're at it, the entire orange family, which should be treated gingerly) and salmon (together with all of the mid-pinks, including Pepto-Bismol and ointment). Don't swallow a catwalk color directive simply because it appears to come from on high. Very often, these things are decided years in advance by a fabric focus group in a Geneva conference room. Your *own* coloring will determine the colors you wear most successfully. Find a palette that you adore, and it will adore you in return. As my friend Tim says, it never hurts to ask if an item comes in a color other than yellow.

5. You do not need a new handbag every season. Sure, it would be nice, but weren't you saving up for a trip to Florida?

WHAT NOT TO WEAR, A QUICK CHECKLIST

In the meantime, do bear in mind that there are some clothes that you should never wear if you want to walk on the skinny side. They include:

* Quilted down jackets
* Belted cardigans
* Oversize knitwear
* Your partner's jeans
* Hot pants
* Tube tops
* Sweater dresses
* Tweed in general; layered tweed in particular

I'd also advise you to think *very* carefully about strapless (particularly on your wedding day). There are about 12 people on the planet who look truly brilliant in a strapless dress, and—love you as I do—I must tell you that it's unlikely that you're one of them. If in doubt, play it safe and pull on a shrug.

6. The only people who look good in capes are superheroes and Mary Poppins. If you are not one of the above, leave well enough alone. Similarly, ponchos are for gauchos. Ditto chaps.

7. A Chanel jacket will not make you thin or beautiful. But it will make you happy.

Armed with this useful list, you will now be able to cut through the Style Lies that litter your life. You will feel free, fabulous, and 5 pounds lighter. Okay, that's a lie. But you might just stop putting leather belts over your sweaters. Small mercies, I say.

50 NEVER BUY CLOTHES FOR THE WOMAN YOU'D LIKE TO BE, BUY THEM FOR THE WOMAN YOU ARE

We all have them, don't we? The Moroccan slippers. The leather pants. The baby-doll dress, the short-shorts that looked so great on Kate Moss . . . all those items we bought for the life we'd *like* to have, rather than the one we're living. My world is thick with impulse purchases for the woman I'll never be: The exfoliating thigh mitt (can't be bothered). The phone that plays music and takes photos (don't know which buttons to press). The white Chanel coat (way too beautiful to wear). The wetsuit (way too ugly to wear).

Even such mavens of style as Sarah Jessica Parker suffer from this Displacement Shopping: "There are so many clothes I want," she said in an interview with *Woman's Day* magazine. "I want more gold cuffs, some great Fendi bags, and anything Nicolas Ghesquière has done for Balenciaga. And of course I want shoes, shoes, and more shoes. . . . And the other thing I can't get enough of is vintage, vintage, vintage. But so much of this is for the woman I think I should be, but the woman I really am is, sadly, going less and less to the shops."

My problem is that I have no problem *whatsoever* going to the shops. When I get there, though, I can quite easily convince myself that there is room in my life for another scarlet lipstick—even though the one I own makes me look like a transvestite and I have never once worn it outside of my own bathroom. The dream is, of course, what gets us out there, trying on a life and buying up a future, even if it's never going to fit. It's how all advertising works—we're sold the idea that we live in a beach house in New England, though it's quite clear that we're stuck in a condo in Cleveland. And so we buy the wicker furniture that would indeed look great on a wraparound porch looking out over the ocean. We stuff it in the family room and hope for the best. The danger is that we spend so much time indulging in a fantasy life, one where we're thinner, wittier, better at diving or chess, that we forget to live our own reality.

The key to dressing thin is knowing—seeing, believing—the state you're in. Thus there are things that I have ushered out of my life because they simply don't work for me. Those racer-back tops that can't be worn with a bra? Hmm. If I don't wear a bra, I frighten small children. The plaid coat? Looks better as a picnic rug. The lovely polka-dot dress that would be a dream if only I didn't own quite such conversational breasts? Out, out damn spots! The point here is that you are not Jennifer Aniston. You are not Catherine Zeta-Jones. You are you. Wonderful, glorious you.

51 DISCOVER WOMEN DESIGNERS

This won't make you fall off your stool in astonishment, but women designers are usually more accommodating of the female body and are therefore worth investigating if you want to give yours an advantage. Most of them admit to designing for their own figures—which is hardly surprising, since that's the body they have to dress every day and the one that's closest at hand in the design studio. Betty Jackson's gentle designs, for example, work well for women who—like Betty herself—want to look taller and slimmer. Donna Karan, one of my heroines and a woman who well knows the value of high-tensile Spandex, refuses to design clothes that can't be worn by a size 12 or 14.

"I'm dealing with the fallibility of a woman's body," Karan once told me. (We were at one of those parties that happen fairly often in fashion— for some reason best known to her publicity department, a vast warehouse had been transformed for one night only into a sultan's pleasure dome. Or perhaps it was a Balinese palace. Either way, I remember a lot of scattered cushions.) "My own shape is rounded," she said, over the din of the 24-piece Congolese drumming band. "I don't have a perfect body . . . show me a woman who does." Karan apparently tests clothes on herself to eliminate gaping shirts and bulging contours and reputedly designs naked in front of the mirror. "I share my secrets with other women," she says. "It's a communication of ways to delete the negative and accent the positive. Let's face it, we all want to look tall and thin. . . ."

Katharine Hamnett, by contrast, started designing precisely because she *is* tall and thin: Sleeves and pant legs were always too short, making her look like an extra in *Oliver!* As Helen Storey—a great designer of the nineties—once put it, "There are bits I can trust, bits I know are familiar to other women. Clothes made by women don't deny what's underneath—we dress the essence, not the male-inspired dream."

So, with female designers, you get no coned breasts, no steel corsets. Not quite so many slut shoes. No bound feet or bustles (Rei Kawakubo and Vivienne Westwood being the exceptions that prove the rule). Women designers—from Stella McCartney to Nicole Farhi, from Vera Wang to Donatella Versace—tend to have known the burden of fat days, bad days, down days, and frizzy hair days. They know the aggravation of that impish squeeze of flesh that escapes a bra. They've probably tucked their shirt into their undies on occasion, or lost a heel to a crack in the sidewalk. While male designers can have imaginations that take them on soaring journeys of creativity, it tends to be the women who know what it feels like when a pencil skirt is cut too tight, recognizing that careful cutting, deft drapery, and an eye on the bottom line are what it takes to dress a woman well. As Diane von Furstenberg, herself an expert at the support and tenderness required to properly furnish a figure, says, "Personally, I have always been attracted to clothes designed by women. Coco Chanel, Vionnet, Norma Kamali, Donna Karan. They have a little more—how do I put it?—*understanding.*" Listen up, sisters. Listen and learn.

52 PRACTICE WARDROBE FENG SHUI

When I moved into my current house, I somehow scored a proper walk-in closet. The sheer delight of *walking in*, pirouetting around, and alighting on today's clever choice of shoe, shirt, or shapewear! You can see it now, can't you? Neat ranks of Manolos, lined up and ready to do battle on my behalf. An entire shelf of color-coordinated cashmere. Boxes of cross-referenced accessories, with an efficient Polaroid index of where and when they last were seen. Ironed pants. How dreamy.

And a dream it is. My friend Lucy stumbled into my "walk-in" not so long ago and fell over a discarded mattress. "Is there a light in here?" she hollered, in a muffled sort of voice that sounded like a small woman trapped under a large mattress. "I think I've stubbed my chin. Is that a lawn mower?"

Lucy had entered The Pit, as this small room is fondly known, in search of a replacement T-shirt for the one her firstborn, Orlando, had just vomited on. Wrist-deep in ketchup myself, and grappling with a child who wanted to stick french fries up his nose, I had gaily waved her off in the general direction of my closet and told her to take whatever she could find.

What she found, it transpired, was an old bedspread, a set of wheeled suitcases, a cup of cold coffee, an original Pucci scarf, and my spare vacuum. (But not a lawn mower. Even I am not that weird.)

Somehow, though, from beneath the chaos, I managed to assemble an outfit each day. An old fashion hack once congratulated me on my inspired pairing of sailor's pants and pussy-bow blouse—little knowing that, like all great works of art, it was but an accident of fate.

Now, though, Lucy was on to me. Oh, the shame. In certain circles, I am considered to know a thing or two about clothes. People turn to me for advice—like the woman who sent me a text message asking for help locating a pair of "elderberry-colored shoes" to go with the table decorations at her sister's wedding. And yet I clearly treated my own clothes with utter disrespect. Shirts were shucked off and left on the floor, where they stayed, neglected, overnight. I had single earrings whose partners had left the building in search of a more sympathetic home. I once moved a step ladder to one side and discovered my black Gucci dress attached to one of its rubber feet. I'd been looking for it for months and had secretly suspected Violetta, our Ukrainian cleaning lady, had taken a shine to it.

And I knew I wasn't alone. Surely, I said to Lucy, the only people with neatly folded clothes are obsessive-compulsives, bored housewives, gay men, and people who work at the Gap? No, she retorted tartly. "You are a wardrobe tramp. You need to feng shui the lot, like Elton John and

Boy George do every so often. It will give you inner peace." And more space for new shoes! I liked the way she thought.

And so, with Lucy in mind, I undertook a wholesale reorganization of The Pit. It took hour upon committed hour, thanks to the sheer mountain of stuff I'd managed to accumulate even while attempting to live a frugal, eco-conscious, streamlined life. Take gloves—I had five pairs of evening gloves. Two pairs of driving gloves. Fifteen pairs of woolly gloves, two pairs of snow-boarding gloves, and a pair of Sasquatch furry mittens from Yohji Yamamoto. I also had 12 pairs of sneakers, plus a pair of bell-bottoms in orange rayon. I still owned a beloved red cashmere sweater that had died years before, tragically, in a terrible hot water accident, and a half-made skirt given to me by Alexander McQueen before he got famous. At the very back of my closet, I discovered six pillows *that I had never seen before*. How could this be?

It wasn't just quantity, though. The whole process of slimming down my wardrobe took forever because I'm a sentimental old fool. Every article trawled from its depths had its own story, its own tale to tell. Here were the zebra-print Dior mules that walked through Hyde Park in the pouring rain. Here the vintage forties tea dress that I wore, incessantly, for 4 months of 1998; I couldn't live without it, until a new model came along and stole my heart. And then there was the hot-pink mohair sweater that I stopped wearing the day I heard P. J. O'Rourke's compelling comment on women's clothes: "Never wear anything that panics the cat."

The funny thing is how tender one feels about past outfits, even though we allow them to lie unloved in the closet, eclipsed by snazzier, sassier replacements. Even now, the smell of my ancient denim jacket—the one that went with me to Mexico and rode horses on the beach at Cabo San Lucas, the one that met my husband on the same day as I did, the one that was lost for a whole week and turned up in the lost and found at the train station—is a Proustian fix. Its warm, comforting tang is my history, its texture my past.

This, however, is no time to play misty. A wardrobe needs to work, hard, in your defense. So get to it. Throw out clothes that no longer fit. Chuck out items that carry a hint of Abba or early Ramones. Rid yourself of anything you haven't worn for 2 years, no matter how painful the parting. I suggest you axe the stone-wash denim, the fake-fur muffler, and anything, however inoffensive, made of corduroy. (If it's vintage, stick it on eBay and reinvest.)

Since my fashion feng shui, I can report that life has become quite a bit simpler. Just having the right clothes available at the right time—a great sweater here, a top there (pressed, and not pummeled to pieces), a blouse that you haven't seen for years but that works like a dream with those cigarette pants—well, it makes dressing a breeze. The consequence is a more considered look and, in turn, a better-dressed you. The consequence of this? Guess what: You've just lost weight.

53 DRESS YOUR AGE, NOT YOUR SHOE SIZE

Okay, in European sizes, my feet happen to be a 39, so the aphorism doesn't quite work. However, the point is that we should really entertain more realistic style crushes as the clock ticks on. It's fine to dress like Lindsay Lohan, Britney, or Mary Kate Olsen if you still live in your childhood bedroom with your menagerie of cuddly toys. But the rest of us would do well to look beyond their miniscule skirts, kooky capes, and midriff-bearing T-shirts, without sacrificing a sense of informed, inspired style.

While fashion pundits tend to be terribly gung ho about the agelessness of clothes, about how the taboos of dress have been broken, and how mother and daughter can now wear the same jeans to the same party where they'll dance to the same tune . . . the truth is that there *are* still boundaries. Not, perhaps, enforced by a society of strictures and codes, but by the fact that a 40-year-old woman wearing lamé shorts looks plain foolish. Youthful clothes tend to revel in the fizzy fact that they are cheap and cheerful, which necessarily means that not a great deal of thought has been lavished on navigating a rounded tummy or catering to heavier breasts.

While midlifers are struggling with the mirror, though, the fashion world remains haughtily besotted with youth, enthralled by its milky skin and pretty feet. For the time being—at least until the fashion industry wakes up to this mature market hungry to spend money on clothes—it's up to you to dress appropriately. Know thyself (you should already be halfway there)—and that elusive word "style" will start to follow you around like a puff of Chanel N° 5.

For a lesson in how to go about it, over to Carine Roitfeld, the 50-something editor of French *Vogue*. Her look (heavy black eyeliner and a wall of hair that threatens to close off her face from public view) is imitated everywhere: on the catwalk, in the weekly newspaper inserts, in the windows of department stores. "Right now," said a recent paean, "Carine Roitfeld is the most stylish woman in the world."

So, Carine? How's it done?

"Leather trousers?" she says firmly. "No good as you get older. . . . For normal woman, with not big money, if I would give advice: Buy mainly classic pieces and a new pair of shoes each season. A Burberry trench coat is always beautiful. Maybe you change the belt and this season you put an Indian scarf." Little things. Big difference. Proper clothes. Slimmer you.

6

HOW TO EAT PETITE, PART II

MASTER THE ART OF CALORIE KILLING

As you will by now have realized, this is not a diet, it's a "live-it," all about simple methods that modify your behavior to maximize your chances of looking like a knockout in that little black dress. I'm not about to demand that you ban cupcakes forever, but the truth is that some fun foods just aren't worth the calories. Banish the ones you don't adore, the ones you could take or leave and only eat because they happen to be sitting in front of you on a nice big plate. Regard the others as special-occasion treats and afford them respect, like you would a visiting dignitary. This chapter examines the what, why, and how of effort-free calorie-slaying. There's plenty of meat on this particular bone, so—rather than feeling overwhelmed by the smorgasbord of choices—cherry-pick what works for you, remembering all the while that this is about enjoyment, not torment. Putting these tips into practice should feel as easy as taking candy from a baby.

54 PRACTICE CALORIE SKIMMING BY ELIMINATING EASY THINGS

And when I say easy, I mean *easy*. Like:

* Removing mayonnaise from your sandwiches (try low-fat plain yogurt, instead)
* Leaving sugar out of your coffee or tea
* Eating sorbet instead of ice cream
* Having a dunk of olive oil rather than a pat of butter
* Switching from whole to skim milk
* Moving from white to whole wheat bread
* Switching from wine to spritzer

See? You'll hardly notice the difference, but your buttocks will. Once those substitutions are second nature, try these:

* Serve crudités, not chips, when friends come over for drinks.
* When you're eating out at a decent restaurant, ask for carrot sticks, not bread sticks.
* Ditch the ketchup. Heinz produces 291,000 gallons of ketchup per day—that's 400 million bottles a year. It is sugary condiments like this that rack up the calories. If you need sauce, make your own salsa with finely chopped tomatoes, spring onions, and a kick of jalapeño peppers.
* Choose fish over meat. And grill your fish, don't fry it.
* Similarly, skin your chicken, trim your meat, and grill it.
* If you must eat beef or lamb, choose "grass-fed" or "pasture-raised" meat: It has significantly less fat, fewer calories, and more omega-3s than grain-fed meat. (These distinctions also imply that the animal was humanely raised.)
* Expand your meat eating to include lean game. Venison, for example, has just 10 percent of the fat found in beef.
* Keep frozen bananas, frozen blueberries, homemade fruit-juice pops, or granita in the freezer instead of ice cream.
* Buy tuna in water; try sun-dried tomatoes that are *dried*, not bathing in oil. If it comes in a slick, say "no thanks."

* Use nonstick cooking spray in your (seldom-used) frying pan.

* Graduate from beef to turkey.

* Have a cheese vacation. (That's a time-out from cheese, not a weekend break at the Vermont cheddar factory.)

* Switch from lattes to Americanos, cappuccinos to black filter. If you're a milk monster, just go skinny (nonfat).

* Sacrifice caffeine altogether if you can, since it is thought to make the body acidic. Develop a green tea habit, instead (see page 118).

* Favor mushrooms over meat: A study at Johns Hopkins Weight Management Center has come to the remarkable conclusion that eating meals made of mushrooms—lasagne, chili, whatever—rather than lean ground beef results in fewer calories being consumed at each meal. Meals made with meat averaged 420 additional calories and 30 additional grams of fat per day. Another study found that if men substituted a 4-ounce portobello mushroom for a 4-ounce grilled hamburger every time they ate a burger over the course of a year, and they didn't change anything else, they could save more than 18,000 calories and nearly 3,000 grams of fat—the equivalent of 5.3 pounds, or 30 sticks of butter.[1] That is a heck of a lot of fat but, one has to notice, quite a lot of mushrooms, too. Perhaps take a modest approach, and make an occasional swap.

* Choose fresh fruit over dried. The drying process concentrates both nutrients *and* calories—which is all very well if you're hiking in the High Andes and don't have much room in your backpack. But on an average day, choose fresh. A cup of fresh apricots, for instance, has around 74 calories and more vitamin C than a cup of dried apricots, which has three times the calories.

* Buy only 80 percent cocoa-solids chocolate. Better still, sleep through Easter and Christmas (or get religion and give up chocolate for Lent).

* Do some research so you know what you're putting into your system. Only 5 percent of people in Starbucks, and 3 percent in McDonalds, bother to read the nutritional information that's available—but it's an easy way to arm yourself with knowledge and make informed swaps. So, in McDonald's, for instance, don't choose a Double

Quarter Pounder with Cheese (740 calories and 42—yes, 42!—grams of fat) when a cheeseburger will do (300 calories and a comparatively reasonable 12 grams of fat). Starbucks' lemon loaf cake, meanwhile, is a deceptive 440 calories a slice; its petite vanilla bean scone is a mere 130.

55 TAKE THE FOOD FACTOR OUT OF THE EQUATION

As actor and comedian Stephen Fry put it, "How did I lose the weight? Prepare to be astonished—I ate less food. That is the only way." There

DRINK YOURSELF THIN WITH GREEN TEA

I well remember the first time I saw model Sophie Dahl, years ago, rolling down a catwalk, all thigh and breast and voluptuousness, barely contained in a cobweb of angora on the catwalk of Irish designer Lainey Keogh. Compared to most of the girls who rattled down the runway, Dahl was vast—a glorious confection of marshmallow, peaches, and cream. We fashion editors loved it, Sophie found fame fast, and then—as if by magic—she shed 35 pounds and three dress sizes. While willpower must have played a strong hand, Sophie herself name-checks the invigorating, fat-busting power of green tea. "I slimmed from a size 16 to a 12 by sipping cups of green tea, which helps to speed up the metabolism," she said at the time of her incredible shrink. This elixir has been hailed as a cancer-fighter, an allergy-slayer, a heart-protector—but all you really need to absorb for our present purposes is that it has virtually no calories and about half the caffeine of coffee. The same goes for ancient Chinese Pu-erh tea, a favorite of Joss Stone and Victoria Beckham. It comes in cake form and needs to be crumbled into boiling water, and it promises to raise the metabolism without stressing the heart. This clever concoction are, however, ways to consume less *and not even notice*. This is the key to nondiet weight loss, the clever way to slim down naturally, effectively, sustainably, healthfully, and (crucial, this) enjoyably—particularly in a culture where food is everywhere you look, waiting to trip you up so you can land facedown in a pecan pie.

Each day, we apparently make more than 250 food decisions. That means we have *choices*. So make the right ones. This applies to all food, whether it's from Les Halles or Le Greasy Spoon. Here's how.

❋ Have business lunches in the office or in a park, not in restaurants with four types of artisan bread and a tempting and comprehensive dessert menu.

apparently burns extra calories without one having to lift so much as a thumb, which means that women—*thin* women—speak in hushed and grateful tones of its capacity to melt fat and reduce cholesterol. But, hey, you don't even need to buy the hype. Just know that a milk-free tea is your drink of choice should you want to shift some baggage.

If you need a little persuasion to tear yourself away from the cappuccinos you're addicted to, consider the fact that chain-store coffees can contain hundreds *and hundreds* of calories per cup. Don't get mugged by a Fattucino; it's time to wake up and smell the calories. (You'll save a fortune, too.)

* Starbucks venti white-chocolate whole-milk mocha with whip, **628 calories** (nearly one-third of your total recommended daily amount)

* Starbucks grande whole milk caffe mocha with whip, **396 calories**

* Caribou Coffee large Turtle Mocha with whip and 2 percent milk, **550 calories**

* Caribou Coffee large white chocolate mocha with whip, **500 calories**

* Caribou Coffee small macchiato, a reasonable **15 calories**

* Starbucks double espresso, **11 tiny little calories**

* Cut down on restaurant visits in general, since you inevitably eat more when dining out (an average of 1,000 calories per meal, and that's not including the platter of mints that you will demolish by accident while waiting to pay the bill). I'm not suggesting you only ever eat at home, by the meager light of a tallow candle. But do think twice before you climb into the car and head off to Pizzeria Uno.

* If you are eating out, do a Bruce Willis: When the star pops into The Ivy, he asks the chef to steam his organic veggies. You may never have saved the world from certain Armageddon, but you, too, can be a bit of a diva in restaurants. This is the 21st century, people, so don't order what they give you, order what you want, and make it lite.

* Ask for sauces on the side, in a neat jug, not corrupting your plate with a puddle of superfluous calories. Do the same with dressing by requesting naked greens and dressing them yourself (with oil, vinegar, and lemon, *not* blue cheese).

* Say "no dessert, thank you" to the waiter *before* he offers you a list that includes amaretto cheesecake, caramel brownies, layer cake covered in chocolate fondant, and three types of homemade ice cream. I mean, really, who wouldn't crumble?

* Squeeze liquid soap on your kids' leftovers. I'm serious—if this is your vice, then slay it now. If a cold chicken finger is beyond your ability to resist, then put it beyond temptation. Make whatever is left on the plate unavailable to nibble on, whether it's with a napkin across the food or, in another radical move, pouring salt over provocative leftovers. It may sound drastic, but it's the picking and the pecking that really piles on the pounds—ask any mother who suddenly has to cope with a whole new meal at snack time. Pretty soon, there's a whole new her in the mirror. As comedian Janette Barber says: "When I buy cookies I eat just four and throw the rest away. But first I spray them with Raid so I won't dig them out of the garbage later. Be careful, though, because that Raid really doesn't taste that bad."

* Wrap tempting tidbits in aluminum foil so they can't make eyes at you through a window of plastic wrap. Nothing looks quite as lonely and in need of rescue as a leftover chicken drumstick.

* Kiss "cook's perks" good-bye—that means no more eating the crusts cut off your children's packed-lunch sandwiches, the "tester" cookie warm from the oven, or cake batter straight from the bowl. This last—despite being an unpromising combination of raw egg and uncooked flour—remains one of the most delicious edibles I know of. Buy a spatula. Scrape all of the batter into the cake pan, not into your waiting mouth.

* If you happen to be in a cafeteria-style restaurant, don't use a tray. Studies have shown that you are likely to fill it up, simply because it's there.[2] Instead, only take what you can politely carry in your hands (holding items under your chin is not part of the deal). In fact, trays are fast being removed from college dining halls across the United States in an effort to tackle obesity and cut down on food waste.

* Studies have shown that if there are lots of options at a buffet, you'll eat more. So only put three things on your plate at a time.

* Okay, so now we're in the realms of mild excess, but if you're an incorrigible dough-head, you need to take action. When the waiter brings bread to the table, spill a glass of water on it. There. That's no longer a threat. Better still, more polite, and infinitely more ethical, ask nicely for "no bread," graduating to "no mayo, no whipped cream, no cocoa-dusted truffles, and certainly no petits fours." When dining out, then, only eat things that are specified on the menu, not all the feel-good freebie bonus bits that will propel you helplessly into a plus-size.

* At home, serve vegetables and salad in heaped, welcoming, help-yourself bowls on the dining table. (This is often called "family style," which is nice. It makes me think of *The Waltons* and gives me a strong urge to bake a blueberry pie.)

* Dole out meat, sausages, mashed potatoes, and other fatteners in individual servings and keep the rest back in the kitchen, out of sight.

* Go food shopping after lunch, not before. A standard supermarket easily becomes a grotto of gastronomic delights if you're starving, thanks to your hunger hormones. I have been known to fall heavily for some vile, prepackaged baked good simply because I hadn't seen

(continued on page 124)

CAKE FEAR: LEARN TO LOATHE THE ONE YOU LOVE

Food, alas, is everywhere. We live in a food soup. And very seductive it is, too. "Food," says Philip Hodson, fellow of the British Association for Counselling and Psychotherapy, "is art, it's decoration, it's interior design. Humans have always used food symbolically, whether in ritual or religion—but now we tend to use it as a drug. It's a love substitute, a sex substitute. If you are touch-hungry, hungry for gratification, eating does, briefly, fill the void. The reason it's difficult to stop eating certain foods is that we're made to feel deprived of what is socially defined as a sensual pleasure."

Remember, then, that food is only and always ephemeral. "It is also," says Hodson, "anonymous: you can love it but it won't love you back." Food, ultimately, is not a solution. It's a means, not an end. So it's time to demote. And, perhaps, time to end a few passionate relationships.

Personally, and I'll admit it's a weird talent, I can spot a slice of lemon drizzle cake across a crowded room. It is a rare meringue that gets past my eagle eye, particularly if it's laden with whipped cream and perhaps a lone strawberry. Chocolate cake actually talks to me, whispering sweet fudgy nothings from under its plastic dome, egging me on, closer, closer, until—*kaboom*—I'm staring at the empty, crumb-filled plate wondering where it all went wrong and whether it would be unthinkable to have another slice. Yup, we all have our soft spots. Winnie the Pooh's was honey. Popeye's was spinach. And mine is proper old-fashioned tea-time cake. Yours might be greasy fries or Amaretto or those molten chocolate cakes that are gooey in the center, as if they have recently fallen in love. Whatever it is, know it. Note it. Now destroy it. How? Easy. Don't let your prime weaknesses through the door: Make a list of the top five foods that make you lose all self-control and send you into a spin of spiraling desire, and prohibit them. Just them. Not everything. Mine are:

1. **Truffled Camembert.** A provocative rendezvous of oozy cheese and perfumed butter that is quite possibly made by seraphim on a cloud far, far away. If it didn't smell quite so much of cheese I would take it to bed.

2. **Lindt Orange Intense dark chocolate.** It knows the way to my mouth without even being given directions.

3. **Doritos.** These delectable triangles come in a vicious orange bag, and—lo and behold!—they are actually vicious orange themselves, coating your fingertips and the corners of your lips with an addictive, radioactive-looking dust. Nutritionally objectionable, but my own Achilles' snack.

4. **Jelly Babies.** Like gummi bears, only cuter. How could you resist?

5. **Butter.** Like my father and my father's father before me, butter is my downfall, my fridge fantasy. I like it on pretty much anything, as long as it's spread thick, a delicious salty slab of sunny delight. I have even been known to countenance the eating of snails once they're coated in this glorious substance.

Right, so there's my list. Yours might include—oh, I don't know—crispy bacon, cinnamon buns, pancakes, wild cherry Life Savers, prosciutto. Whatever your Fat Five, treat them like vampires and don't invite them in. Sail past them in shops, give them the cold shoulder at parties, bitch about them to your friends. We're not in the business of martyrdom. I'm not about to suggest that you eat dry toast with a knife and fork while staring longingly at the jam. But let's be fair here: If you are banning *just* five fattening things, there's still plenty of room for treats—just not the ones that will fill your head, your heart, and your favorite jeans. I find that a simple swap for a less-loved alternative will cut consumption in half. Unsalted butter has, for me, none of the seductive appeal of the salted stuff; standard Camembert is far less interesting than the truffled variety; and I'm safe from the pull of Lindt, as long as I avoid the Orange Intense flavor.

a calorie since breakfast. Go after lunch, and you'll be far more circumspect in your purchases. (Take PMS into any store, at any time of day, by the way, and you'll come out with chocolate.)

* If you *do* come out with chocolate, break off two squares and put the rest away, repeating to yourself: "Nothing tastes as good as being thin feels" in a voice like Dorothy in *The Wizard of Oz*. Beware, then, the Proximity Principle: A study conducted at the University of Illinois used Hershey's Kisses to show how having food conveniently close makes you eat a whole lot more of it. When workers kept the chocolate on their desk, they ate an average of nine Kisses per day; when it was moved just 6 feet away, they ate only four per day.[3] This is your cue to remove temptation. Don't give yourself the choice of whether to eat the nachos or not; just don't put the nachos on the table. Better yet, don't buy the nachos in the first place.

* Similarly, keep sugar in a bag, closed with a clip, housed in a Tupperware container with "Keep Out" stenciled on the top in Sharpie. In the shed. Don't have it in a bowl, placed a convenient distance from your elbow.

* Just cook *enough*. Not too much, but enough. Being of Italian descent, I generally make twice the amount of pasta recommended on the package, in the belief that too much is always preferable to too little. I invariably end up with great steaming vats of farfalle, pans brimming with fusilli, linguine as far as the eye can see. I then compensate for my profligacy by subjecting the plates to overfill. Pasta slips, slops, and spills over the edges and, quite often, onto the floor, all voluptuous and glossy and fetching. I proceed to eat as much as I can (no, no, not off the floor!), like one of those hicks from the sticks in a chili dog–eating contest. *Disaster.* The way to navigate this calorie pit is to avoid it completely. Cook less. An average portion of rice or pasta for an adult is ½ cup. Cook just this amount and you won't have to mop the floor so often, either, so it really is win-win.

* Be the last at the table to start eating, and the first to stop.

* Remember that leftovers are all the more delicious (somehow) for being surplus. This is an oddity of food: It is so much more appealing

when it's somewhere other than on your plate (on your partner's plate, for example). The gooey deliciousness that lurks under a cooling roast chicken needs no introduction from me—and while it should perhaps remain in your world as an occasional treat, on the whole, try to defend yourself against the leftovers before they coo and woo. Either produce the right amount of food in the first place, or wrap up any extras and get them out of sight directly after serving. A cooling plate of roasted potatoes eyeing you while you're drying the pots is a dangerous thing indeed.

56 PRACTICE PORTION CONTROL: POLICE THE FOOD ON YOUR PLATE

"If you buy a cookie at a [train] station," says Tim Lobstein, PhD, of the International Obesity Task Force, "it's 4 inches across! Compare that with the [cookies] your granny used to eat. Companies are selling to our eyes rather than to our health needs. And it's only if you read the small print that you can tell what's going on."

It's true that there has been a portion explosion in the last 2 decades, leaving us facing vast heaps of food at every turn, armed only with the vague notion that it is polite to finish up everything on a plate. In their study of why the French remain so much slimmer than Americans, researchers from the University of Pennsylvania came to the remarkable conclusion that it was because the French ate less. The figures—both physically and statistically—back this up. Average portion size in Philadelphia was about 25 percent greater than in Paris. A supermarket soft drink in the United States was 52 percent larger, a hot dog 63 percent larger, a container of yogurt 82 percent larger. A croissant in Paris weighs 1 ounce; in Pittsburgh, it's 2.[4]

Surveys show that one in four Americans eat everything they're served, no matter how enormous it may be. The United States is indeed the land of giant pastries—although New York City's Board of Health voted unanimously in March of 2008 to require all city chain restaurants to post calorie data on their menus, which may well serve to bring ballooning portions back down to earth. A fascinating study at the University of California's Center for Weight and Health showed that Californians could avoid gaining 2.7 pounds a year if calories were featured on fast-food menus statewide.[5] Knowing how many calories are in your Venti Mocha Frappuccino may well give you pause, or even embarrass you into ordering an Evian.

It's certainly worth a try. I well remember being overwhelmed by the sheer girth of a muffin I once bought at a coffee shop in Brooklyn—but I braved my way through it under the wayward assumption that it constituted a "portion" and therefore ought to be finished. This, I later discovered, was a classic behavior known to psychologists as Unit Bias. "If food is moderately palatable," says Paul Rozin, PhD, one of the researchers on the Pennsylvania study, "people tend to consume what is put in front of them, and generally consume more when offered more food." Interestingly, hamsters do much the same thing.

In another experiment by Brian Wansink, PhD, at Cornell, subjects were placed in front of a bowl of tomato soup and invited to drink as much as they wanted. Unaware that the bowls were being filled covertly from below, a surprising number of people kept right on drinking until the experiment was halted. Was this bottomless greed? Stupidity? Or simple human instinct? Revealingly, Dr. Wansink also showed that even *nutritional science professors* ate 50 percent more if served in bigger bowls and with bigger spoons.[6]

The issue, then, is that our environment is encouraging idiotic gluttony. Even our glasses have exploded, happily holding three servings of Merlot and still leaving it room to breathe. In certain restaurants, the wine vessels are virtually impossible to lift without mechanical assistance. Tiffany's top-selling wine glass now holds an extravagant 15 ounces, which is more than enough to send me nose-diving into the salmon appetizer.

The solution?

✳ Think small, delicious mouthfuls from small, pretty plates.

✳ Use your senses. Think, taste, and smell while you eat.

* Leave packaging and food detritus on the table, in the manner of a Dionysian feast, so you can see at a glance how much you've consumed.

* Use tall, thin glasses (we tend to pour more into short, fat ones).

* When in doubt, buy smaller spoons.

* Dining out? Sit opposite a mirror. Eating in? Install one behind your breakfast table. Go subliminal.

* You could do worse than remember the *Sex and the City* mantra: "Order fashionably. Eat sparingly."

* Check the packaging: Does the lasagne box say "Serves Four"? Is it trying to tell you something? Do not forge ahead and eat the whole thing in one gluttonous sitting. And do try to remember that the nutritional information on the back may refer to a single serving, rather than the whole thing. If it says "Only 15 calories!" in alluring yellow letters on the front of the package, look hard until you find the revealing disclosure that this is "per serving."

* Decant food into a small and delightful receptacle, rather than eating it straight from a box, bag, carton, or tub. Put all tubs away in a distant cupboard.

* When serving food, leave what great Japanese chefs call "a margin of emptiness" at the edge of the plate; this is, says renowned chef Masaru Yamamoto, the "emptiness of an aesthetic significance, comparable to that in Zen ink painting." That's reason enough to do it, in my view.

* Listen up: You don't have to eat everything on your plate. Really, you don't. "Clean your plate" is what exasperated mothers drum into their preschoolers. Unless you are wildly precocious, if you're reading this book, you are not a preschooler. Start taking control of your plate.

* Know when to say when, and then say it again.

* If you crave seconds, live with that thought for a few minutes, allowing your stomach to catch up with your mouth. After 10 minutes, you're less likely to want the extra spoonful, no matter how lovin' it looks.

* Buy, make, and serve individual portions. So, one toffee, not an entire pan of fudge. One cup of sorbet, not a vat of vanilla. A handful of

chips poured into a single-serve bowl (a ramekin would be ideal), not one of those bags designed for sharing with extended family at a barbecue.

* Cultivate Tupperware Pride: Collect useful receptacles in which to chill or freeze leftovers, rather than going for seconds simply to clear a plate. Look upon this as the good, honest, labor-saving, planet-loving, flab-busting endeavor that it is. Label well. You don't want to end up with nameless containers of unidentified matter in the netherworld of your fridge.

57 IDENTIFY WHAT'S IN YOUR TAKEOUT

Takeout food is, in general, loaded with calories. Fast food is fat food, so think very carefully before you stroll through the golden arches or pick up the phone. Bon Appétit!

TAKEOUT	FAT CONTENT*
Au Bon Pain Turkey and Swiss Sandwich	41 g
Boston Market Pastry Top Chicken Pot Pie	47 g
Burger King Whopper and large fries	69 g
KFC Crispy Caesar Salad (with Creamy Parmesan Caesar Dressing and croutons)	48 g
McDonald's Big Mac and large fries	54 g
McDonald's Chicken McNuggets (10 pieces)	29 g
Long John Silver's Battered Fish (2 pieces) with small fries	42 g
Panera Bread Sierra Turkey Sandwich	40 g
Pizza Hut Supreme Pan Pizza, 2 slices	32 g

The recommended Daily Value (DV) of fat is 65 g or less based on a 2,000 calorie diet.

58 READ *FAST FOOD NATION;* YOU MAY NEVER BUY A BURGER AGAIN

"The food revolution of the 20th century was quite remarkable. How food is grown, cooked, processed, marketed, branded—all this has changed utterly in the past 25 years or so. Because we have lived through it, we aren't amazed by it . . . "[7] So says Tim Lang, PhD, professor of food policy at City University, London, and the man who years ago first brought "food miles" to public attention. To fully appreciate your diet—and by that I mean the stuff you eat, not the stuff you *don't* eat in order to lose weight—you need an awareness of where it comes from, how it came to be, and who benefits from its production and sale. Raising your consciousness by knowing the story behind your food, from farm to fridge to fork, or (possibly) from lab to lunch, will serve to halt your hand as you reach for another Tater Tot.

Today, despite years of reeducation, realization, and reassessment, plenty of food still comes from places that don't remotely resemble farms. If you wander around in the center section of your supermarket, you'll see that little has changed, regardless of the traceability and sustainability arguments that rage on at the periphery. I once had a friend whose job it was to "invent" meat products. We would sometimes sit in a bar coming up with new versions of mechanically reclaimed protein with which to tempt the market, starting with a snappy name, a packaging proposal, and an advertising tagline. Alas, he was not the man behind the Slim Jim or any such golden goose, but we did spend a good deal of time chortling about the obvious appeal of "Meat Feet" and "Chicken Lips," which, as far as I know, never quite got to market. Things may be improving, but we do still have "Potted Meat Food Product" containing "partially defatted cooked pork fatty tissue." Now, I'm not suggesting that this is part of your average daily intake—not knowingly, anyway. But plenty of processed foods contain suspect ingredients, massive doses of salt, and high levels of saturated fat. So think about who really benefits from turning potatoes into waffles and cheese into string. Diverting as they may be, such products are nutritionally corrupt; to digest them at all, our bodies must find the missing minerals, vitamins, and enzymes elsewhere—a depletion that, cruelly enough, makes us feel *even hungrier* as our bodies signal for us to replace the nutrients we lack.

Your best defense is to ask the right questions and read the right books, and never again will you be tempted by fake foods. Along with

Fast Food Nation, by Eric Schlosser, try *In Defense of Food,* by Michael Pollan, and *Not on the Label,* by Felicity Lawrence. You'll lose weight and gain wisdom.

59 NEVER BE HUNGOVER OR STONED

These are the fastest routes to fast-food joints and the fridge.

60 DROP THE POP

We all know that Diet Coke is for fat people. But so is regular Coke. Aim for no more fizz, no more "soda" (such a benign word for such a fiendish thing), and none of that organic elderflower pressé, either. Drink water. From a tap. If the tap doesn't turn you on, buy a water filter. Thrill yourself with a slice of lemon, the clink of ice cubes, and the thought that it's virtually free. Yes, you have to grow accustomed to the (lack of) taste— but once you do, it's all you'll want.

As you drink, you might like to dwell upon the fact that our taste for diet drinks could be partially responsible for our current obesity problems. Counterintuitive as it may seem, recent research suggests that consuming zero-calorie sweeteners *increases* the risk of putting on weight. Circumstantial evidence is already convincing: Over the past 2 decades, the number of Americans who regularly eat foods containing sugar-free sweeteners has doubled, while obesity levels have skyrocketed. But now scientists at Purdue University in Indiana have set about analyzing the link. In studies, they found that rats fed yogurt sweetened with saccharin (a sugar substitute) ate more, and grew fatter, than those eating yogurt sweetened with glucose (the real thing).[8]

The researchers posit that sweet foods provide an "orosensory stimulus" that suggests to the body that a deluge of calories is about to come its way. Like Pavlov's dogs, we've learned that sweet, dense, and viscous foods promise lots of lovely calories. When, as with diet drinks, the advertised calories don't materialize, the system becomes confused—and as a result, "people eat more or expend less energy than they otherwise would," says the journal *Behavioral Neuroscience*.[9]

If that's not enough to put you off drinking yourself silly on zero-calorie soda, consider too that processed diet foods and no-cal drinks tend to replace fats and sugars with synthetic alternatives and lab-designed nutrients, some of which are known to be toxic. *Toxic!* This is, needless to say, cause for alarm. And the nondiet alternatives? Packed with sugar. Bad sugar. Fructose—the type of sugar that is found in fruit but is also added to fizzy drinks as corn syrup (because it's cheaper than sucrose or glucose)—is more likely than other types of sugar to cause fat to be deposited around your middle. Because fructose is metabolized differently than other sugars, it is also turned—at startling speed—into body fat.

There's a size issue here, too. In an attempt to boost their profit margins, many fast-food restaurants have taken to eliminating smaller drink sizes and adding ever-larger sizes. A new study suggests that this policy has led to a 15 percent increase in the consumption of high-calorie drinks—since humans, in all our semisentient glory, tend to avoid the smallest and largest options when ordering soft drinks, no matter what the volume of that drink may be. Thus the demand curve shifts ever upward. "People who purchased a 21-ounce drink when the 32-ounce drink was the largest size available moved up to the 32-ounce drink when a 44-ounce drink was added to the range of drink sizes available," say the authors.[10] This means there's a real risk that at some point you'll find yourself watching a movie accompanied by a 7-Up that requires its own seat. Tsk. So many reasons to ban the can. (Did I mention burping? Or the markup on Pepsi? Or your teeth? Do I need to?)

61 ARM YOURSELF AGAINST CALORIE AMBUSH

Your social life is chock-full of opportunities to binge. Be prepared by following these fail-safe rules.

At a Cocktail Party

* Eat beforehand if you can; otherwise, the canapés will beguile you with their beauty and charm. Pre-eating will also soak up any alcohol coming your way, allowing you to leave the room with decorum and without falling over the doorman.

* If you *have* to eat at the party, go for high-protein canapés. Try asparagus wrapped in Parma ham, smoked salmon on Pumpernickel, mozzarella and cherry tomatoes, shrimp with a zingy lime dressing. Feel free to eat the low-fat pretzels and anything you find floating in your drink (olive in a martini, mint in a mojito, celery stick in a Bloody Mary).

* Steer clear of cocktail sausages, even if they are all seductive and sticky with honey mustard. They are cute but deadly—the hippos of the cocktail scene. Similarly, avoid nachos and their wicked posse of high-calorie dips; also buffalo wings, *foie gras*, pizza fingers, and anything made predominantly from cheese.

* Don't station yourself by the swing door to the kitchen in the hope of snapping up the nibbles before anyone else has a chance. This is a well-trodden path toward an elastic waistband.

* Don't follow the waiter around the room, no matter how fetching he may be.

* Don't hover over the canapé platter. It looks desperate and spreads germs.

* Don't pick up more than you can hold between finger and thumb. (One finger, one thumb.)

* Don't let the waiter top up your flute. Go to the bar. Walk there. Better still, tap dance across the room. Work for that drink.

In a Bar

* Nuts are high in fat and are usually salted. The peanut picking that so easily accompanies a gin and tonic is the very enemy of thin, so go without.

* A few olives are okay, if you must.

* Tapas, by the way, is still food, even if it comes free with the beer at an authentic Spanish restaurant. Proceed with caution.

AT A PICNIC

This outdoor delight remains one of the few meals still revered in our culture, which is reason enough to indulge. Rushed as we are to eat breakfast on the go, to do lunch in 3 minutes flat, to get dinner out of the microwave and onto the table, much as we have pushed food to the outer extremes of our lives, the picnic still demands reverie. Relaxation. It's a time to linger, to graze. But there are ways to keep a lid on this idyllic form of calorie consumption.

* Don't rely too heavily on beef and pork products, those age-old staples of the picnic blanket,

* Take smoked salmon (with a bit of cream cheese and dill), turkey breast (a great source of low-fat protein), hard-boiled eggs with coarse kosher salt, and some imaginative greens.

* Widen your repertoire with—oh, off the top of my head—toasted couscous, roasted pumpkin, some exotic fruit, or some good soup in a Thermos.

* Plan it well. Prepare your food in advance, rather than just buying it all en route to the park. You'll have a lot more control over what goes into your food—and your face—that way.

AT A BARBECUE

It is an irksome fact of life that just as the weather demands that you unveil yourself to all and sundry, the barbecue season begins in earnest. The traditional meat fest—particularly if undertaken every weekend from mid-June to Labor Day—will leave you looking like a prize-winning bull.

* Instead of burgers, sausages, ribs, and wings, go for kebabs with a 60:40 veggies-to-meat ratio. Stick some zucchini, mushrooms, peppers, tomatoes, and onion on there instead of all that meat. (For the record, carrots don't work.)

∗ Go for grilled shrimp, corn on the cob, tuna steaks, a whole fish—bass, trout—baked with dill and lemon juice in a foil pouch.

AT CHRISTMAS

Oh, come on! It's Christmas! Live a little. Eat a lot. But do it for one day only. Two, max. The problem with the festive season is that it lasts so very long, stretching further each year, that soon there won't be a point in taking down the decorations. Christmas has, as a result, become a gargantuan eat-a-thon. Little wonder that the pounds rack up. The way to stop the glut and the gluttony is to contain Christmas. Let it run amok, but only for a day. Here's how:

∗ Anticipate festive excess by eating sparingly the week before; that way, you'll be working from a deficit, allowing you to splurge with a happy heart.

∗ Keep in mind that fruitcake, Christmas cookies, turkey and all its attendant trimmings should be shoveled in on the Big Day itself, with leftovers for the following day. Don't start on the Christmas nosh just because your child has appeared as third donkey in the Nativity Play. Last year, the Nativity Play at our school was on November 13th.

∗ Don't overbuy, confusing profligacy with hospitality. Go for quality over quantity. And savor, don't devour.

∗ Don't eat foods "invented" for Christmas—this includes gingerbread in the shape of Christmas trees, mulled-wine flavor cashews, and chocolate spiked with gold, frankincense, and/or myrrh.

∗ Don't keep snacks stashed around the house, telling yourself that you've got them there in the event of guests. Your mouth is allowed to be empty for part of the festive season, so don't cram your life with additional snacks, whether they're bowls of nuts, dishes of toffees, dates, walnuts, yogurt-covered raisins, or chocolate Santas. Hang delightful wooden ornaments on your tree, not cocoa solids.

∗ Remove all Christmas edibles from the house on December 27th. If you can't make a nutritious soup from it, get rid of it.

AT A ROMANTIC DINNER À DEUX

You don't need me to suggest that you eat moderately. The very act of dining with a potential new boyfriend is a diet on a plate. (If only you could have one at every meal.)

* I can confidently predict, but I'll remind you anyway, that there will be no sizzling fajitas, no rib racks, no great tureens of linguine. Basically, you don't want stuff that squirts or dribbles, or anything that requires you to tuck a napkin into your bra. All of which is good from a calorie-cutting perspective.

* Don't go thinking that ordering tempura is an act of the coquette. It's deep-fat frying, no matter how you dress it up.

AT A CHILDREN'S BIRTHDAY PARTY

I know, I know. There is something exquisitely provocative about the uneaten pizza crusts your child has abandoned in favor of Musical Chairs. And I have great difficulty handing around the Oreos without popping a whole one into my mouth and shutting it ever so quickly, like a trap door, leaving me momentarily unable to answer simple questions, such as "Who ate the last Oreo?" Hard as it is to accept, though, stealing food from the mouths of babes is just not okay.

* If you must do it, steal the celery sticks and the baby carrots, which are generally in plentiful supply.

* Try to avoid having "a chip," "a cookie," or "a small handful of M&Ms." There is no putting the genie back in that bottle once you've uncorked it.

52 BAN TRANS FAT

I have always been proud of my Italian heritage. I like the fact that my great-grandfather was a Florentine milliner called Cesare, a man who would apparently rub raw garlic on a hunk of bread for breakfast and who doused his food in olive oil when the rest of Britain was still only using it to dislodge stubborn earwax. I like that my grandmother went by the name of Norma Maria Gabriella Annunciata Maranghi, a billowing breath of a name, undulating, lilting, like a swallow flying over the Ponte Vecchio. I love that a small but significant part of me sprang from a country that might not be great shakes at governing itself or keeping tabs on the paper clips, but that was so very interested in shoes and handbags and wine and food and art and love. In short, all the good things in life.

Needless to say, an Italian—ancient or modern—would never consider eating many of the processed foods we salad-dodgers consume today in such quantity. There's not a lot of love in artificial cream, no great joy in a dehydrated soup. But you will find other things lurking in there. Like trans fat.

These hydrogenated vegetable oils (HVOs) are unsaturated fatty acids that manufacturers use to give texture ("mouthfeel") to food and to help preserve it. As Maggie Stanfield points out in her book *Trans Fat*, "Invented fats of this type are—like natural fats—absorbed into our cell membranes. They fill the space that healthy fats should occupy. . . . Once the trans fat is in position, it cannot be rejected so the integrity of the cell is compromised. The entire behavior of the cell alters and this tiny link in the chain of human life, this miniature cuckoo, is empowered to disrupt the whole natural pattern of biological exchange between cells."[11]

All right, you say, but do they make you *fat*? Stanfield argues that "it may be that we store trans fat more efficiently and easily. A highly regarded study carried out in North Carolina showed that, even with similar calorie intake, trans fat increases weight gain."[12]

As of July 2008, the city of New York has banned artificial trans fats from its restaurants—and if a city of that size can do it, then you can, too. A vociferous and effective campaign against trans fats means that they are fast disappearing from supermarket shelves, but they're still there in many branded products, including sweets, stock cubes, frozen meals, cookies, pastries, cereal bars—even vitamin capsules. Since January 2006, food labels in the United States have had to state trans fats quantities. Even so, your best bet is to wean yourself off "invented foods" altogether. If you fancy going hardcore, avoid anything with a long shelf life. You are, after all, not leaving on a 2-year excursion to the Antarctic. Your food doesn't need to withstand a nuclear holocaust. The market is just up the street—so freshen up and stop opening quite so many hermetically sealed pouches and vacuum-packs. It has been estimated—possibly by a bored student compulsively eating Twinkies—that the average person in the West eats over 4 kilos (about 8 pounds, 13 ounces) of food additives every year. To properly redress the balance, go old-school. Look for fresh food that's full of life. Rubbing raw garlic on a hunk of bread for breakfast is, of course, optional.

53 READ FOOD LABELS. BETTER YET, USE YOUR COMMON SENSE

In a cruel and startling irony, it turns out that plenty of the "healthy" edibles available on our supermarket shelves are no better than the standard full-fat versions. The British magazine *Which?*, in one of its regular investigative forays, found that a low-fat Oreo has 50 calories, while a regular Oreo has 53 calories. This news is thoroughly depressing and likely to drive you straight to the snack cupboard in desperation. (Come on, I know you've got one.)

Most of us already recognize that the modern food shopping experience is beset by the constant drone of worry: *Are we eating enough mackerel? Does mackerel contain mercury? Are there (gulp) any mackerel left in the sea? Wasn't there something about not eating wild? Or was that farmed? And isn't Jemima allergic to fish anyway? But does she eat chicken? And is free-range better than organic? But isn't it a bit unimaginative to serve chicken at a dinner party these days? Shouldn't it be sea trout on a bed of microgreens? Is it too early for a glass of wine? How can it only be quarter to four?*

So here we are, burdened with information and really none the wiser. In fact, as the practice of nutritional labeling on foods has expanded, *so have our waistlines.* Info-load—far from galvanizing and arming the consumer in the pursuit of health—seems to encourage many of us to tune out. My favorite example of this state of affairs comes from lawyer Giovanni di Stefano, who recently got a bee in his bonnet about Kit Kats: "Do you remember the Kit Kat?" he said, "The chocolate bar? Today, when you get the Kit Kat, it says 'open here.' ARE WE THAT STUPID THAT WE CAN'T OPEN A PACKET OF KIT KAT? If we need someone to tell us, 'please open Kit Kat here'—*porca miseria, siamo arrivata allo Massimo!* [hell's bells, we've reached the limit!]"[13]

Quite.

In order to assist us in our search for good nutrition, the Food Standards Agency in the United Kingdom is considering the adoption of "shock tactics" similar to the warnings on packs of cigarettes. Dairy snacks, for example, might be emblazoned with graphic images of clogged blood vessels and fatty deposits. These images will have to be placed somewhere alongside the Ingredients List, the chart showing the Percentage of Recommended Daily Allowance, the Serving Suggestion of the food within, the UPC code, the warning list of allergens contained within . . . by the time you've worked your way through all that, you'll have missed lunch and be hurtling toward supper, questions bouncing around your empty belly.

So, while label-checking is a worthwhile and noble endeavor, don't become a small-print geek, consumed with anxiety and turning food into a trial, not a triumph. If you mull over the nutritional—not to mention the ecological, social, and global—significance of every purchase you make, you'll be stuck in the aisle for weeks, paralyzed under the fluorescent lights until someone wearing a polyester tunic mops the floor around you.

What you really need is a bit of plain common sense and a couple of trigger words that should make you smell the coffee and change your mind.

* Make sure your supper is mostly food, not mostly numbers. Would your ancestors recognize what you're eating? Great. If they'd run a mile to avoid it, you should, too.

* Avoid clearly alien foodstuffs—"extruded starch food products," for example. Shun obvious enemies such as high-fructose corn syrup,

BEWARE CALORIE CREEP

When the nutritional information from a decade ago on a dozen leading brands was compared with today's numbers, nine showed an increase in calories, sugar, or saturated fat. Researchers found that Kellogg's Rice Krispies contain 36 more calories per 100 grams now than they did in 1983—an increase of about 10 percent. Häagen-Dazs Belgian Chocolate ice cream contains 16 percent more calories than it did in 1994 and 26 percent more fat. Even products marketed as healthy options are not immune to this "calorie creep." Experts say the findings, derived from a comparison of current labels with old ones stored in museum archives, fit a pattern whereby manufacturers remove salt and some types of fat from food for health reasons, only to compensate with sugar and more fat. "Reducing salt is an excellent measure, but as a result companies are faced with bland processed food," explains Tim Lobstein, PhD, former director of the Food Commission and now head of the child obesity program at the International Obesity Task Force. "The cheap way of flavoring it up is to sugar it. Fat can also help because it helps your tongue notice the flavors—that's why you butter bread," he said.[14]

The message here is simple enough: Despite best intentions, food labeling is not immune to spin. Make sure that you are.

fractionated palm kernel oil, partially inverted sugar syrup, and partially hydrogenated vegetable oil.

* Don't buy anything where the carton weighs more than the product. As a basic rule, if there is more here to throw away than to eat, it's out. If it's dressed like a prom queen, it's out. If you can't tell what it is by looking at it, it's out. If you have to use pliers to get at it, guess what? It's out.

* Food—glorious, marvelous food—is pleasure, not poison. Love it, enjoy it, savor it.

64 WAKE UP IN THE SUPERMARKET

Shopping for food used to be a rather routine and enjoyable exercise. Stroll to corner shop; request pound of ground beef; inquire after Ethel's sciatica; pay; return home to mangle the potatoes or beat the children. It could happily take all day, what with the chatting and the mangling.

These days—though many of us would dearly like to spend entire Wednesdays wandering around a farmers' market on the lookout for lavender scones and locally raised lamb—the inevitability is that we'll end up in the supermarket. We'll be lured in by lavishly labeled frozen pizza and instant potatoes, by mayonnaise in a squeeze container and boxes of cheap wine.

Yes, a supermarket is convenient and economical and sometimes there's a lady in there giving out free samples of lemon meringue pie. But it's also the native habitat of overprocessed convenience food, and it is designed to suck you in and spit you out in the parking lot, having just purchased three-for-the-price-of-two New York–style cheesecakes.

Today, 88 percent of our food comes from supermarkets, and the very fact that there's so much food, all there, under one vast roof, glinting in its shiny wrappings, simply encourages us to buy (and consume) more. Shopping for food has become a homogenized and strangely hollow experience. On the whole, we're divorced and detached as we purchase our weekly stash—and it is this limited, truncated relationship with food that can be so destructive. Consider for a moment the way we shop at those supermarkets: Having first stowed our brains in the trunk of the car for safe-keeping, we amble about, alighting on items that seem familiar, falling for the sorcery of modern marketing, blinded by gaudy packaging and deafened by the insistent beep of the barcode scanner. Research shows that up to 80 percent of our decisions are made subconsciously as we patrol the aisles. When questioned, some shoppers couldn't remember picking up certain items or didn't know why they had bought them.[15]

Recent studies of the shopping subconscious conclude that many people find shopping a chore, so they tend to switch off and act on autopilot. People armed with a list of 10 things usually bought 60. "Of the visual stimuli that assail a shopper," the study found, "typically only 1 percent makes it into the brain's sensory buffer store, and of this, only 5 percent gets to short-term memory, where it may be matched with previous experience and/or advertising to trigger an emotional response." It's all a bit Orwellian, isn't it?

So wake up. Right now. Stick to a list. Ignore Two-fers and BOGOFs on Chips Ahoy! If you continue to shop at your favorite supermarket—and I don't doubt that it's easy, reasonable, comforting, and relatively painless (unless you're doing it with toddlers in tow)—do try to do it with *awareness*. Your bottom line will benefit, in every sense.

55 PUT THE PLATE IN ITS PLACE

If you dream of donuts, it's time to find something better to feed your fantasies. Look, it's great if your glass is always half full, but if you talk about nothing but eating, discussing lunch at breakfast and dinner at lunch, then it's time to switch your attention to something more edifying. Here's how to turn yourself off to switch yourself on.

* Meet friends for a walk in the park, a jog in the gym, a book club, a back rub—rather than at your favorite coffee shop. Your mouth needn't be full to be having fun.

❋ Wean yourself off TV cooking shows. The Food Network is there to inspire, not to suck you in for hours, until it's bedtime. If you watch a program on how to make your own pumpkin and pine-nut ravioli, dressed with pesto and crispy sage leaves, and then you stir yourself from the couch to open a can of Spaghetti-Os, you're missing the point of it.

❋ Fear not an empty fridge. "I think that it goes back to the rise of the big American fridge," says food writer Joanna Blythman. "It's an aspirational thing." Indeed it may be, but having great truckloads of Cheddar, whole hams, and four-tier coffee-walnut cakes littered about the place is the highway to the wide way. You don't want a completely empty fridge, of course, but aim for something that inhabits the happy middle ground between Spartan and wanton, perhaps containing just enough to see you through a snowstorm.

Once you start to think about food in a realistic, rational way, you'll begin to see that you can modify your behavior around it. You can even playfully push it out of the way. The following hints may seem a trifle silly, but they worked for me.

❋ Discover a fingernail in your favorite brand of muffin (or imagine that you have). Something similar happened to me with a particularly delicious sandwich of chicken, bacon, mayo—the works—that I had become accustomed to eating every other day at lunchtime. One day, halfway through this fat fix, I bit into something rubbery. Bacon? *Eeeew,* chicken skin? I rolled it about in my mouth. My mouth was perplexed. On examination, it was a bandage. A bandage! In my mouth! Never. Never. Never. Again.

❋ Choose things on the menu that you don't fancy much; it will broaden your palate and your horizons, not your waistline. I once did this with crispy pigs' ears in London; I have also done it with snail porridge, ducks' hearts, and pigs' tails in various other places, frogs' legs in New Orleans, and stir-fried locusts in a back alley in Bangkok (having just had a tattoo of a new moon etched on my shoulder). The point is to view food as an experience—not as comfort, crutch, or custom.

This investigative, alert relationship with supper is what you're after. Which reminds me of two quotes—one from the philosopher Ludwig Wittgenstein (who apparently said "I don't mind what I eat, as long as it's always the same thing," so the great man was clearly a ninny); and the other from Parliament member Tony Benn. Benn wrote in his diary that he has a thing about Triple Cheese Pizzas, and has "eaten two of them every day for years." Good grief. I want to take the poor man out for a plate of crispy pigs' ears. Rather than settle for the same-old, try instead to take your taste buds on a journey they'll never forget. Besides, if it's locusts for lunch, you're guaranteed not to want seconds.

* Ignore free food. This includes samples at farmers' markets, chocolate that comes through the mail, food served on sticks at conferences, unexpected bonus courses in upscale restaurants, that half of a muffin your friend couldn't quite finish . . . fat traps, all of them.

* But for heaven's sake, don't get super picky. Try not to panic if a cream sauce arrives with your fish. A spoonful of sin does not a lard-ass make. Better, by far, to have friends.

56 BEWARE "SALARD" AND OTHER HIDDEN FOOD TRAPS

While dodging obvious calorie hazards, it's equally important to avoid apparently "healthy food" that has been dressed to the nines: "salard," for example—defined as a meal that starts out green, good, and leafy but soon becomes heavy with cheese, egg, bacon bits, croutons, shards of Parmesan, Thousand Island dressing, and some leftover chicken wings, all loaded on board in a bid to jazz it up. Similarly, just because the words "pasta" and "salad" happen to meet on the side of a takeout container, it doesn't mean that the container actually holds a salad. It is *cold pasta.* With mayonnaise, flecks of tuna, and an afterthought of chopped red pepper. Just as a gym membership card alone will not make you fit, so a meal containing broccoli will not make you thin. Use your brain and stop lying to yourself.

But before you head off for the salad bar like a beatified martyr, you may also like to consider this: According to a series of studies at Cornell University, "the 'health halos' of healthy restaurants often prompt consumers to treat themselves to higher-calorie side dishes, drinks, or desserts than when they eat at fast-food restaurants that make no such health claims." The findings, published in the *Journal of Consumer Research*, reveal that people also tend to underestimate by up to 35 percent just how many calories so-called healthy foods contain.[16] The answer is to go easy. Don't cram. And don't award yourself a Snickers as a prize because you've had a chicken wrap that contained grated carrot. I know you. I'm watching.

67 DRINK LESS ALCOHOL

It's 8 p.m. End of a long day. Traffic jam. Tax man. PMS. IRS. Irritating acronyms. Irritating husbands. That guy in front of you at the bank who was exchanging his pennies for dollars. Sheesh, it's no wonder you're tired and frazzled. The sofa is all set to give you a hug. But first? First, you'll open a bottle of wine.

Of course you will. We all do it. That nightly bottle of Shiraz or Chardonnay has become the comfort of a generation. Most women I know spend regular evenings in with Ernst and Julio Gallo, occasionally flirting with an audacious Robert Mondavi or some exotic import. Our grandparents, you may remember, drank wine, if at all, as a treat. They may have had sherry on the sideboard, a gin and tonic in the backyard, and sweet liqueurs, all sticky labels and crumbling corks, available for the resuscitation of elderly visitors. But they didn't have wine by routine, night in, night out, with barely a night off.

Plenty of us do today, though. So now is the time to bid the bottle *adieu*—not forever, but perhaps just Monday through Thursday. Instead of having a nightly blowout on cheap wine, come home to a simple omelet, a pile of deep-green spinach, and a single glass of really good wine. Something to savor. You'll gain so much—and here's what you'll lose: the morning headaches, the groggy half-sleep during breakfast, the dehydrated mouth on the ride to work, and the 10 pounds that have settled around your middle like a lazy pet dog.

It's well worth doing, for more reasons than one. You see, the increase in alcohol consumption among females has apparently caused us to accumulate weight less around our bottoms (be grateful for small mercies), but more around the middle, similar to the traditional beer belly on men. You don't need to be told that this is not a good look. Nor is it a healthy one. And while the health implications should give us all pause as we reach again for the corkscrew, the weight factor is perhaps more immediate and compelling. We'd do well to sober up and face the facts before we're all built more like beer barrels than wine glasses.

IN THE DRINK: HOW MANY CALORIES IN A BIG NIGHT OUT?

Alcohol has around 7 calories per gram, making it twice as fattening as protein or carbs and almost as calorically dense as fat. Interestingly, a martini has about the same number of calories as a slice of cheese pizza. Calories in a drink are sad and "empty," being of no earthly value to your poor beleaguered body, apart from making it feel momentarily irresistible. You'll know the truth by daybreak, trust me.

DRINK	CARBS (G)	CALORIES
Beer (12 oz)	13	140–160
Red wine (4 oz)	2	85
Gin (1 oz)	0	65
Tequila (1 oz)	0	65
Vodka (1 oz)	0	65
Whiskey (1 oz)	0	64
Lemon juice (1 Tbs)	1.3	4
Lime juice (1 Tbs)	1.4	4
Orange juice (4 oz)	13.4	56
Tomato juice (4 oz)	5.1	21

All drinks were not created equal, so it's time to crack down on the fatteners and go slim. Luckily, some spirits—tequila, gin, and vodka—contain no carbs. That is not to say that they contain no calories, but it does mean that they are preferable to downing great vats of vino, which can really add up, if you're not concentrating. Clearly, the very point of alcohol is that you soon stop concentrating, allowing you to wander the streets late at night falling into hedges and singing "Danny Boy" to the lampposts. In weight-loss terms, this is hopeless. Drinking not only inhibits sleep, it stimulates appetite (which is surely the only reason the 24-hour diner persists in our culture). Nutritionists recognize that the body processes alcohol before it gets to work on fats, proteins, and carbohydrates—which means drinking slows down the burning of fat. Worse still, it reduces inhibitions, allowing you to do crazy things, such as finding out how many M&M's you can fit into your mouth at one time. Hilarious, yes, but not helpful if you're aiming to fit into that bikini anytime soon.

Bear in mind, too, that a glass of wine used to be one serving; now—thanks to those generous glass sizes—it's two. If you insist on having a drink, here are a few pointers.

* Stop drinking dry white. Start drinking vodka (but not in the same quantities).

* Keep adding ice cubes.

* Sip. Don't gulp.

* Choose small glasses; fill them halfway, in the manner of a top-flight sommelier.

* Keep the opened wine bottle in the fridge or in a seldom-seen cupboard so that, should you wish to refill your glass, you need to set out on an expedition.

* If you *have* to snack while drinking, avoid salty stuff: It makes you thirsty so you drink more (which is why every bar serves peanuts or pretzels).

* Educate your mouth: Train your palate to appreciate fine wine and reject appalling swill. Buy one great bottle and savor it.

* Make every other drink water.

HOW TO MIX THE PERFECT DRY MARTINI

If you *are* going to indulge, make it something memorable. Something glamorous. Something like a martini. The marriage of gin and vermouth is not only classically chic, it is an alchemy of flavors that is entirely magical. How could a pizza compete? Here's how to do it right.

* Ignore Bond's advice. A dry martini *must* be gin-based; vodka is inert in the presence of vermouth, which leaves you with nothing but a mouthful of boredom.

* Keep your liquor in the freezer to ensure that everything is sub-zero cold.

* Pour a hint of vermouth into an ice-filled shaker. I said a hint. Not a slosh. Connoisseurs call for $\frac{1}{15}$ of the quantity of gin you intend to use. I prefer $\frac{1}{7}$.

* Stir. Don't shake. Honestly, 007 really was a double-oh-ditz when it came to martini-making. (Shaking adds way too much water and obscures the point of this drink.)

* Discard the vermouth; enough of what you need is clinging to the ice.

* Add your chosen gin and a drop of Angostura Bitters, if you're that way inclined. Stir again and serve.

* Watch your mixers. Club soda, lemon, and lime juice are your best bets; orange juice will double the calorie count of a vodka shot.

* Stop drinking irresponsibly. No more reds with chicken or fish!

* If, like me, you're in the habit of pouring yourself a very generous glass of Pinot Gris as soon as your children are snoring gently in their beds, you will get through a serious number of servings over the course of an average week. Introduce Teetotaler Nights—say, Monday through

Thursday—when you lay off the booze completely. You could halve your weekly alcohol intake this way; you'll also slash your liquid calorie consumption, wake up with a spring in your step, cut back on your shopping bill, and—if you're anything like my friend Dan—start that novel you've always been meaning to write. Personally, I have taken up the piano and now play "Für Elise" on such a loop each evening that I am annoying the neighbors.

7

THE ART OF ILLUSION

DIVERSION, DISTRACTION,
AND DECEPTION

So here we are at the heart of the beast. You've already made brilliant progress by eating well, engaging more, judging less. Excellent. Now it's time to fake it. These canny moves, gleaned from my years in the fashion industry, will unveil the slim new you in seconds, without any need to deny yourself a decent lunch. You'll discover ways to shave off an inch here, a bulge there; ways to run interference so that your assets get all the attention and your liabilities sneak under the radar; ways to fib and flatter so you'll never need to diet again. Once you've tried them, you'll love them for life. Here, then, are the tricks of the trade.

68 WEAR HEELS. ALWAYS

"Good heavens!" said my father not long ago, shocked enough to keep his espresso hovering just below his lower lip. "That is the first time I have ever seen you wearing flat shoes!"

He wasn't being strictly accurate, of course, unless I sprang from the womb wearing a nice pair of Manolo Blahnik slingbacks. (Anything is possible, I grant you, given my lifelong predilection for heels.) I do believe I wore flats to place third in the 100-meter dash in 1976, and again to climb Mount Snowdon by mistake in 1992. (We took the wrong path in the mist and arrived at the summit entirely by accident. I had thought I was popping out to buy a granola bar.)

But, in principle, my dad was right. I am indeed rarely out of heels. There are people I have known for years who have no idea how tall I really am. I have worn platforms on the beach at St. Tropez. I have driven for more hours than I care to remember in a finicky pair of complicated stilettos. My feet are so used to living at a 45-degree angle that I feel giddy on flat ground, like sailors must feel when they're getting their land legs.

In this respect, I am much like Victoria Beckham, who apparently "can't concentrate in flats." (Though my all-time favorite quote on the subject comes from Mariah Carey, who says, "I can't wear flat shoes. My feet repel them.") From our lofty perspective, there is no earthly point to a flat—why, I asked my lanky friend Veronica, would you want to slap through life, your feet flapping about like Olive Oyl's, when you could teeter and totter about like a foal?

"Because," retorted Veronica, "Women in stupid bloody heels look vaguely incapacitated at all times, as if midswoon and expecting a man to leap to their defense."

She's not keen on being manhandled, Veronica. But she has a point. The wearing of high heels is perhaps the last bastion of unreconstructed antifeminism left in our wardrobes, and one that many of us embrace so willingly. Yet we all know that high heels hurt. They send our hips forward (if we're walking like a catwalk queen) or our asses out (if we're not). They compromise our spines and trash our very soles. They are hazardous to ankles. They ruin hardwood floors. Proper high heels, incidentally, are also fiercely expensive. But still we love them so.

We love them because they are a shortcut to sizzle. Superlative shoes can add sex to any outfit, regardless (and this is the crux) of the body that sits on top of them. They also trick the eye into believing that your legs are longer than they are, making you look instantly thinner. In my fattest, darkest moments, a pair of Sergio Rossi tomato red slingbacks has dragged me from the depths. When I was pregnant and built like a prizewinning pumpkin, Manolos got me through. As most canny women know, vertiginous heels are the fairy dust that turns jeans into dynamite, tailored trousers into rock 'n' roll cool, pumpkins into princesses.

For Nicole Kidman, a woman of 5 feet 10 inches who was forced into humbling flats for the duration of her marriage to Tom Cruise (5 feet 7 inches), heels meant liberation. "Now I can wear heels," she sighed as their divorce came through, and what she meant was, "Now I am free." For others, they mean "Now I am rich." Look at Elizabeth Hurley, Victoria Beckham, and Paris Hilton, their feet routinely housed in non-shoes made from angel breath and unicorn hair, proclaiming to onlookers that they never have to walk very far. Interestingly, Victoria Beckham wears those strappy shoes way beyond the red carpet: She wears them to attend football games, to traipse through airports, to stroll the world's prime retail acreage. She wears her glass slippers long after the ball; she wears sandals in a snowstorm. Today, bizarrely, this is the mark of the prodigiously rich.

A shoe, then, is no mere afterthought: Whether you are with the upper crust or on the lowest rung, it is the basis of your day, plotting the curve of your spine and the wiggle in your walk. (I need hardly remind you that Marilyn Monroe had her Salvatore Ferragamo shoes made with one heel lower than the other, to lend that reckless roll to her gait.) There is, when you stop to stare, so much cargo in those meager scraps of leather, so many messages transmitted by tongue and sole. If you get your shoes right, right now, then you're part way to dressing thin, and you haven't even pulled up a zipper yet. Next time you sling on your shoes as you rush for the door, choose with care. Choose a heel. Lose a pound.

THE DOS AND DON'TS OF SHOES

Footwear is no afterthought. It is the very basis of smart dressing and your platform for change. Some shoes will cleverly, graciously whittle away the weight, while others will only add to your excess baggage. It pays to know precisely what a shoe can do for you, so accompany me now on a journey through the highs and lows of heels.

Slingback. The most seductive of shoes, chiefly because the strap is ever perilously close to collapse, leaving you—*swoon*—naked from the ankle down. They're a bit careless, slingbacks, and thus hopelessly sexy. They also have an illusion going on, leading the eye all the way from hem to toe without any troublesome obstacle, unlike the . . .

Ankle strap. This, by some freak of design, will effectively chop your legs off before they're finished. Needless to say, this is absolutely not advisable if you're after a long, lean look. Wear only when they're at the very peak of fashion (for about 10 minutes every third year). Otherwise steer clear and go instead for the . . .

Gladiator. Yup, the ancient shoe that wouldn't die. There is something very appealing about a whip of leather pirouetting up a shin. Reminiscent of a corset, with a mild fetish overtone, gladiators—flat or high—manage to make a calf look contained, and thus slimmer, avoiding the ankle strap trap by encouraging the eye ever up rather than stopping it dead in its tracks. What's more, gladiators that chase up a leg manage to disguise a multitude of sins (varicose veins, stubble, unsightly blotchiness). All good, I hear you cry, throwing down this book to get your mitts on a pair. Well, yes . . . but first a word of warning: Do beware of the sun. Lattice-striped shins will make you look like a garden trellis, which is almost as bad as a . . .

Round toe. Why? Because a stumpy toe can easily steal an inch or more of height from your frame. Add an ankle strap, and you have the world's most fattening shoe. Apart from the . . .

Ballet flat. Worn with the wrong clothes, the ballet flat wins the contest for "least slimming shoe." I have one pair of red flats that my husband calls my "fat shoe," which somehow takes the shine off wearing them. With a full skirt they make me look several sizes wider. They do, however, look marvelous with capri pants, a marriage made in style heaven, as dear Audrey Hepburn demonstrated so prettily. My most treasured ballet pumps are silver, which only adds to their allure. (I'm debating the purchase of the gold, which might just be too much, like having solid gold faucets in your master bath.) Anyhow, the rule is to wear ballet flats with slim-fit pants—cigarette pants, capris, skinny jeans, that kind of thing. Wear them with a short, full skirt, and it's curtains. What you really need with a swishy skirt is a . . .

Kitten heel. These darling shoes manage to walk the tightrope of making your feet look adorable and petite, while allowing them to perch on a reasonably low, stable heel. This is a plus for any woman who actually has to walk between engagements. They are, however, one of those styles that tiptoes into fashion from time to time, rather than being a constant companion. If kitten heels don't seem to be in fashion this season, settle instead for a . . .

Pointed toe. Oh, do I really need to tell you how vampish and gorgeous they are? Not ideal if they are out of fashion, as is occasionally the case, but they truly triumph when they are trendy. Go for a toe that could puncture tires and a heel that promises death to all invertebrates foolish enough to cross your path. Wearing them regularly may, of course, make your feet look like they've been beaten with a rolling pin. But what the hey! Pointy-toe shoes care little for comfort. They rock, they roll, but they certainly don't buy you flowers inquire about your health. They do, however, manage the dual feat of elongating the leg *and* slimming the ankle, while giving passing men the impression that you will not take it lying down. A similar effect may be obtained from a . . .

(continued)

Peep toe. To my mind, though, this other leftover from a bygone age ought to be stamped out, chiefly (though inexplicably) because it gives the strong suggestion that you have just stubbed your toe. The peep toe is also faintly silly, a design detail too far. Why does your middle toe need a sunroof? If your feet are hot, wear . . .

Strappy sandals. Yes, they are the preserve of the super rich, worn by the limo classes, women who have the soles of their shoes polished. But still. In her book *I Want Those Shoes,* Paola Jacobbi says, "Look at sandals—they are the bikini of footwear . . . you can be fully dressed but in some way you are naked; you can wear strappy sandals and your whole look is subverted. That's why women will wear them even when it is cold or they have to walk far." The rule here is to wear them only if you have decent feet: No corns, bunions, warts, calluses, or any other objectionable features. If your feet leak out between the straps, please return them to the tissue-lined box and opt instead for an . . .

Ankle boot. These little pixies have been hogging the limelight lately, and with good reason. Half-shoe, half-boot, the versatile hybrid waltzes through the seasons like there's no tomorrow. My own favorite is the "shoot," the result of a midnight encounter between a shoe and a boot, resulting in a crossbreed that looks perfect under pants and still manages to walk the walk with tights and a skirt. On the whole, however, anyone with generous calves really ought recognize that an ankle boot will make them look like Nellie the Dancing Elephant. Far better to go with a . . .

Knee-high boot. There is, after all, something dashing about a really great boot. Flat riders, bikers, cowboys, piratical, slim, zipped, elasticized . . . it matters little what you choose. These heroes will cradle your legs and steal an inch or more from their circumference. If you can't find a boot to fit, try a Web site such as Zappos.com, which has a wide selection in different calf and foot sizes. If it's height you're looking for, though, you'll want to look for a . . .

Platform. Hopeless when you're in a hurry, but a perennial favorite. I have loved them for decades. My very first platform shoes were bought for me during that long, hot summer of '76. They were easily as long as they were tall, decorated in flower-bedecked cotton and impossibly dangerous for a 9-year-old child to negotiate. It was like having a couple of pocket dictionaries attached to my elementary-school feet—and even today, I am amazed that my mother (who made me wear two pairs of pants on cold days) allowed me to have them at all. Still, a love affair started then, and to this day I'm a fan. Platforms, you see, are a great way to add length without the demanding tightrope walk of a proper stiletto. Bear in mind that they are, by nature, blocky and can easily make you seem bottom-heavy, strapped to the ground like Neil Armstrong to the moon. Avoid enormous stack heels of the kind that could unwittingly flatten small children. If in doubt, try a . . .

Wedge. Again, you'll acquire the illusion of stature with less wobble than with a skinny heel, thanks to a broader, safer center of gravity. Perfect for the navigation of grass, uneven sidewalks, the lawns of country clubs during wedding receptions, and cobblestone streets, and significantly more interesting than the . . .

Pump. There are several ways to go with this one. Play it safe (navy, mid-height, block heel) and you will look like a government worker. Not that there's anything wrong with that. But if you are on the hunt for a little *ooooh*, a little *aaaah*, and a whole lot of thin, you'd do better to raise up and slim down that heel. Always avoid fat heels. Fat heels = Fat feet. Black and navy shoes are, incidentally, about as interesting as . . . as . . . yawn. Sorry, too bored to even come up with a simile. Let's move on.

FIND YOUR WAIST AND CHERISH IT

And so to the tricky issue of high-rise versus low-rise waists. It's one of those perennial issues of fashion, and you'll already know which camp you prefer. But are you doing yourself any favors? Should you reconsider?

First, a word in favor of high-rise pants. Nicole Kidman looks absolutely amazing in them. She looks like a sapling, a human exclamation

BABY, BABY, WHERE DID YOUR WAIST GO?

In 1941, the average American woman had a 27-inch waist. By 2004, according to SizeUSA findings, it had expanded to 34 inches—that's around an inch a decade, and counting. This points out the intriguing paradox that while we are desperate to keep up with our ever-shrinking celebrities, the average woman is getting wider. (You know this already if the old romantic in you has ever tried to cram itself into your grandmother's wedding dress.) "Women resemble men much more so than they did in the fifties," confirms Jennifer Bougourd, senior research fellow at the London College of Fashion. "While we are bigger overall, the waist has grown more, in proportion. Modern women are very much straighter now."

Quite why this is happening may seem obvious: We eat too much. But it's not just about quantity. Says Emma Stiles, nutritional scientist at the University of Westminster: "The waist-hip ratio has changed over the last 100 years because of a change in the macronutrients in our diet. Our intake of carbohydrates and sugars has grown rapidly, which increases insulin production. This in turn aids fat-cell deposits on the torso rather than anywhere else on the body." It turns out that while our celebrity icons threaten to slip between the cracks in the pavement, the rest of us can barely slip through a turnstile. If we resemble anyone these days, it's not Posh Spice. It's Elton John.

mark. If anything, they make her look taller and more elegant than she already is. And this woman is *tall*. She makes Kate Moss look like a footstool. On such a slender ribbon of a thing, the effect of a high waist can be dynamite.

For those of us burdened with a belly, high-waisted pants are, by stark contrast, nothing but a blight. If, like me, you are more curve than taper, they will do you no favors at all, apart from, perhaps,

How, then, to deal with this thickening? Eat less. Sure. But you can cheat, too.

* Pick out designers who really know how to throw a curve at a woman's body. Roland Mouret, for instance. His long-loved Galaxy dresses, and many of his more recent creations, are underpinned by a canvas, boned "waist restrainer" with a metal-toothed zipper up the back for support.

* A wide belt will do the job of a corset if you find the latter a bit too hard-core.

* A wrap dress, a ballet cardigan, a wide sash tied in a bow like a Christmas morning surprise? All great ways to make your waist work and leave your bottom out of things entirely. An obi sash or a wide belt will perform the same magic.

Another way to fake it is by working not on your overall shape, but on your proportions. "Modern women are looking at the waist-lines in the magazines and thinking, 'How am I going to wear this?'" a fashion buyer once told me. "To create that tiny waist today, given our new proportions, you have to cheat, by giving volume to the skirt and cropping the jacket higher." Got that?

keeping that roly-poly tummy of yours warm in a draft. Should you insist on taking part in this trend, however, here are some tips. Number one: Always wear high waists with high heels. Exquisitely high heels that require you to sit down often. Number two: Make sure your high-rise pants are made from a slimming fabric, not the kind of tweed that thickens you until you look more trunk than sapling. And number three: *Breathe in* if someone threatens to take your photograph.

Your alternative is to stick with the groovy rock 'n' roll lounge look of low-rise pants, which can do much to elongate a dumpy, stumpy sort of figure. Mind you, low-slung has its issues, too. Butt cleavage, for one (*hello moon!*), which is frankly rude in mixed company, or the ludicrous sight of a thong peering out above a waistband, as if looking for predators. Sarah Jessica Parker, herself an arbiter of style and a skinny little thing to boot, told *Vogue* some time ago that she doesn't consider low-rise pants to be age-appropriate for a woman such as herself. It's up to you to make that choice, but do bear in mind that alighting on your waist and making a fuss of it is one sure-fire way to catch a dose of the slims.

70 MASTER OPTICAL ILLUSION AND THE TRICKS OF *TROMPE L'OEIL*

There's so much to remember. I suggest you photocopy this bit and stow it in your handbag.

* A V-neck will lend your body a subtle vertical line. This is good.

* A turtleneck, though, will make you look like a turtle. This is bad.

* A plunge neckline (particularly a loose cowl) can flatter a bigger bust (if you give it enough alcohol).

* Flared legs will balance fuller tops. (That's pant legs, not *your* legs.)

* A shrunken jacket makes everything look smaller—but not if your bottom is vast (see next two items to remedy this problem).

* If your bottom is wide, a drop-waist skirt will minimize it.

* An A-line will work to make your bottom appear smaller, chiefly by leaving it alone. But be aware that an A-line can easily turn into a tent. Try before you buy.

* To elongate a figure, loop a long, filmy, printed scarf—not a fat cravat—around your neck.

* Extreme heels will slim an ankle. Duh.

* A long necklace, à la Coco Chanel's pearls, will lengthen the torso and enhance cleavage.

* A wide belt can help keep a tummy under control. Not too tight, mind you. It shouldn't look uncomfortable.

* A high-waisted skirt in a supportive fabric will streamline the tummy (as Nigella Lawson will confirm). The trick here is to wear your heels and your collar high to create a sinuous, endless silhouette.

* Chokers will slim down a medium-size neck. But note that chokers will choke a very thick neck. Let your mirror (and your ability to breathe) be your guide.

* If you have heavy thighs, an empire line—belted or ribboned—can accentuate your narrowest part. Do this. Do it now. Beware, however, the unfathomable pull of the baby-doll dress. An empire needs to be sleek and assured. It should not suck its thumb and ask for a lollipop.

* A front crease in tailored pants will elongate the leg; back pockets will slim a big bottom.

* Pleated pants are suspect (at least if you want to look thinner). The additional fabric adds bulk and makes you look like the keyboardist from any number of 80s bands. Go for flat fronts, which keep everything nicely tucked in.

* Pants with cuffs tend to shorten the leg.

* Black shoes with black opaque tights will make your legs go on for miles. Ditto tan legs and nude shoes.

* If your body is blocky, try a contrasting mid-panel; a long scarf or a black jacket over a light-colored tee will perform a similar trick.

* Floaty layers are usually kind to bulges. Don't go too frou-frou, though, or you'll look like a Portuguese man-of-war.

* Velvet and corduroy tend to thicken a body by reflecting light. (You'd get the same effect from wearing carpets.)

* Similarly, shiny fabrics make you look bigger, which is why cyclists should wear them and women in search of elegance should not.

* A two-piece, two-color outfit—your skirt navy and your jacket beige, say—is horrible. It will skew your proportions and incite a fight between your upper and lower halves. When planning an ensemble, go for something that elongates your figure, taking the eye on an exquisite journey from halo to toenail, *not* something that chops you up like a magician's assistant.

* A twin set, however, has an absolute *gift* for optical illusion: The shell clings to your frame (great), while the cardigan offers camouflage, comfort, and shelter in a stiff wind. It also distracts the eye from an ample belly. Brilliant. Be patient; they'll be back.

* If you have pockets, keep them empty. Seriously. What earthly point is there in buying expensive handbags (which I urge you to do—it's just such *fun*), if you insist on keeping your cell phone, your lipstick, your shopping lists, and a coin purse in your pocket? A full pocket is like a full diaper: objectionable in the extreme.

* I like this tip from fashion designer Sir Paul Smith, a man who knows a very great deal about successful dressing: "If you have a big bust, stick to single-breasted blazers to avoid adding volume. Longer-line jackets flatten rounder hips. High heels, rolled-up sleeves, and pretty jewelry will stop this look from becoming too masculine."

* And this, from fashion designer Betty Jackson on dressing curves: "To find your ideal summer dress, look in a mirror at the area between the collarbones. Anything that drapes, knots, tucks, crosses, or folds along that vertical body line (be it high or low neck) will disguise problems brilliantly—particularly if it's flattened down by stitching. These design details will shave off inches while allowing ease of movement and look really elegant."

THE UPS AND DOWNS OF STRIPES

A word about vertical stripes. I know—dull, dull, dull, but they work . . . or do they? In a spot of sensational myth busting, psychologists at York University have found that vertical stripes are more fattening than horizontal ones. In the study, volunteers looked at 200 pairs of images of women in several sorts of stripes. Horizontal stripes were judged significantly more slimming (to make the women in the pictures appear to be the same size, the ones wearing the horizontal stripes had to be 6 percent wider).[1]

Peter Thompson, PhD, who led the research, is mystified as to how we could have gotten it so wrong, pointing out that scientists have been aware of the unflattering properties of vertical stripes ever since German physiologist Hermann von Helmholtz created his "squares illusion" in the 1860s. Von Helmholz drew two identically sized squares and put vertical stripes on one and horizontal stripes on the other; the square with the horizontal stripes appeared taller and thinner than the other square, prompting Helmholtz to note that "ladies' frocks with cross stripes on them make the figure look taller."

In truth, stripes of any persuasion can be challenging. Though chic, they distort in a very obvious way when navigating a bulge, which is a bit like drawing an arrow on your belly and asking people to throw it commiserative glances. If you're keen on wearing stripes, go with the brilliant sailor-top classic, or widen the stripes for a punky punch. Do avoid vertical candy-stripes, though, particularly around Christmas, when you might be mistaken for a candy cane.

71 WEAR INTERESTING AND DIVERTING ACCESSORIES

* If at all possible, buy diamonds.
* Otherwise, go for thumping great accessories—like those vast handbags and sunglasses worn by Paris Hilton, Lindsay Lohan, and

Victoria Beckham. Not only will you look thinner, but you'll also burn calories as you lug it all around. Genius. So good, in fact, that *Marie Claire* was prompted to call the idea "one of its top diet tips for summer." (You can achieve the same dwarfing effect with huge DJ-style headphones, roller skates, or a very big boyfriend.)

✳ Never embellish a problem area hoping to disguise it. You may as well draw a target on your butt and invite onlookers to try for a bull's-eye. If you have an ample chest, avoid breast pockets and double-breasted jackets. If you're wider than you'd like to be, steer clear of side pockets and overskirts, unless you're auditioning for a role in a Britney Spears video.

✳ Bows, frills, and ruffles are *not* interesting and diverting accessories. They ought to be confined to your kids' dress-up clothes, or at the very least conferred upon someone who might find them useful when filming period dramas, such as Keira Knightley. My great aunt Betty, a substantial woman in every sense, habitually wore flamenco frills, most often in the colors of international flags. She forever looked like a galleon in full sail or a pair of Austrian blinds cruising up the hallway en route to the nearest Whitman's sampler. If fashion dictates ruffles, find your inner anarchist and tell fashion where it can go. Quote Leonardo da Vinci to shore up the argument: "Simplicity," he said, "is the ultimate sophistication." (See diamonds, page 161.)

✳ Stall the audience at ground level. Blissfully, most design houses have gotten into the swing of producing shoes crazy enough to be certifiable, which makes them both conversation pieces and a terrific diversionary tactic. Shoes are becoming more and more ridiculous, as if afflicted by a cumulative condition that will one day send them over the edge in a flailing hail of sequins and snakeskin. Choose from the feathered, mirrored, and patent; go for color, texture, and tantalizing heel shapes. If Prada's hand-sculpted shoes don't keep the eye off a bountiful bottom, I don't know what will.

72 KNOW THE ENDURING STRENGTH OF BLACK

Now I recognize that it's not fun with a capital F, but if you really want to slim your booty, the very best way to do it is to discover the enduring power of black, navy, and, to a lesser degree, neutrals. Dull? Possibly. Dense? Fair point. Effective? Hell yes.

Despite criticism that wearing black tends to weigh down a figure and disguise curves—breasts, for example, which can be a delightful addition to a silhouette—the bare fact is that black is a thinning agent. If you transport yourself for a moment back to the physics lab of your past, you'll remember that white reflects light and makes things look larger (think of a room); black absorbs light and make things look smaller. Yippie-ki-yay! Johnny Cash was really on to something, as Peter Thompson, PhD, psychologist at the University of York, confirmed in a recent experiment: "Wearing black is a good thing," he concluded. "That one works. We looked at a black circle on a white background and a white circle on a black background. The black circle looked smaller than the white one."[2]

It is this reliable optical illusion that perhaps explains why a recent survey found that 41 percent of our wardrobes are made up of black clothes. Each of us, on average, owns five black coats, two little black dresses, and 12 pairs of black shoes. No wonder our partners rarely notice if we've been out on a shopping splurge; marvelously, it really *does* all look the same to the untrained eye.

I checked my own wardrobe against these figures—breaking down my formidable closet into color-coded zones, a bit like the parking garage at Ikea. I was amused to discover that 70 percent of my wardrobe is resolutely black, and a further sizeable chunk is navy-blue, which is little more than a coy excuse for black. On the shoe front, from sneakers to towering stilettos, I own 36 pairs of black shoes. I found, to my astonishment, that I actually possess two identical pairs of black ballet flats, which I have been wearing for 3 years thinking that they were one and the same pair. And as for little black dresses? My evening wardrobe has relied for so long on the forgiveness and chivalry of black that I can lay claim to only three posh dresses that contain any color at all—and one of those was bought for a costume party when I (unfathomably) decided to go as Elizabeth Taylor in *Who's Afraid of Virginia Woolf?* The rest is black to the bones.

Since this tends to look funereal, as if all your clothes have gathered for a wake, it is worth spiking it up with jolts of color, flashes of flesh, and the occasional print, if fashion and climate allow.

73 GO FOR LOW-KEY PRINTS: BUSY PATTERNS WILL MAKE YOU LOOK LIKE A SOFA

Have you ever entered a room—a party, perhaps, or a gathering of some sort—and had a stabbing feeling in your soul that people might think you've come in costume? It's one of my personal dreads, and I have spent all my years in the fashion game trying to walk the very thin line between looking enviably trend-aware and going an inch too far and looking like the hired entertainment—a trumpet player, perhaps, in the samba band. Play it too safe, of course, and everyone will overlook your dress sense entirely and concentrate instead on other things you might be good at, such as whistling. Play it too wild, and those same people will whisper about your fondness for galoshes the moment your back is turned.

It's a tricky balancing act—in fact, it's the very heart, the art, of fashion itself—and it's made all the more complicated when the fashion for "fun prints" rolls around, as it does every fourth summer or so.

These vibrant prints are delightful, of course. I love them all: Those splashy florals that greet you like a slap in the eye with a cold washcloth, the naive doodle prints, those blocky geometric ones that are very MOMA. All of them are crazy and cool. *But* they are all, without exception, teetering right on the brink when it comes to that line between incredibly wow and hopelessly whoops. Splashy prints take up twice the visual space of their more restrained cousins. They add weight, and they cause a fuss. If people take one look at your outfit and say any of the following, you're in trouble.

* "Why have you come dressed as a pizza?"
* "I had a throw pillow like that once."
* "Don't be mean, she's wearing it on a bet."
* "Whoa! You've spilled chicken casserole all down your front! Oh, you haven't? It's the new Vuitton print? Gosh, awfully sorry."

If pushing for a print, then, here's what you need to know to avoid looking like a hot-air balloon.

* A small, subtle print on a dark background will shed weight.
* Big ethnic or graphic prints can disguise lumps and bumps (think tribal).
* While stripes of any variety are not flattering to an ample figure, geometric patterns and organic shapes are. They serve to break up the area covered, confusing the eye into believing it's smaller.
* Delicate florals are, on the whole, kinder than wild, devil-may-care swirls. Laura Ashley was not wrong. Well, not *entirely* wrong.
* Keep your prints under control: A scarf (Pucci, Gucci, or Hermès, perhaps) will confine your pattern to a nice contained space, like mint in a flower pot.

74 DISCRETION IS THE BETTER PART OF GLAMOR, SO KEEP YOUR MIDRIFF UNDER WRAPS, EVEN IF IT'S FLAT

I don't want to sound like an old fogey, but most naked midriffs are about as attractive as most naked bottoms. They loll over a waistband, like a neighbor over a fence. They bulge at the sides. They pucker at the back. Even though fashion has, strictly speaking, moved away from the midsection to focus on greener pastures, they're still all over the place, littering the landscape like so many spare tires. I saw a girl on the bus the other day whose midriff virtually had a life of its own; I half expected it to lean over and say, "Nice weather we're having, don't you think?" or suggest an answer to 9 Across.

To my eye, even those rare toned tummies are mildly vulgar, a private place carelessly on parade. Ditto the small of the back, that low-rent lodging place for trampy tattoos. The fact is that a slim and stylish woman simply doesn't flash too much flesh, and even the flesh that *is* flashed needs to be treated judiciously. Take, for instance, the upper arm. That unassuming zone, which until now has meekly gone about the duty of joining your shoulder to your elbow, suddenly turns on you when you hit your midthirties. Suddenly entire sections of your wardrobe are obsolete: the tank tops, the tiny tees, the tube tops, bra tops, camisoles, and vests. Whole species, wiped out.

Some of us, of course, are more likely to suffer this loss than others. My fate, alas, is written in my genes, thanks to an Italian grandmother whose upper arms would swing happily in the breeze at summer picnics. I remember being hugged by those warm panels of flesh, a place that smelled of security and lavender water and a peppermint lost in a handbag. Which is all very well if you're 79 and have trouble remembering where you put your glasses. At my age, when you're still considering a Spanish beach vacation and have long glossy hair and good ankles (did I mention them?)—well, slack triceps are nothing but a trial and a tribulation.

The solution lies in the cut of your tops. Sheer sleeves will mask chunky arms. Flippy sleeves on summer tops go a good way toward distracting the eye while retaining adequate ventilation. Don't think, though, that you can divert attention from your wings by showing off your midriff. The world doesn't work like that.

8

ON BEAUTY

HOW TO DISGUISE FLAB, FLUBBER, BLUBBER, AND BLOAT

Most people, most of the time, are looking at your face. Promise. You may think that it is your grand expanse of a backside that is soaking up all of the attention, but more often than not it is your eyes, your smile, and your hands that will captivate an audience. Beyond all that, there are ways to buff up that body and make it work for you. All you need is the know-how.

75 MAINTAIN YOURSELF!

Style—though as much in the knowing as the doing—does require a certain degree of effort. Unless you are built like Cate Blanchett or you're under the age of 18, you can't simply tumble out of bed and hope for the best in the belief that yesterday's makeup is somehow very Patti Smith circa 1978.

So maximize your chances. Make the most of what you've got and you'll feel leagues better . . . feel better, and you'll look better. Simple, really. It's all about maintenance—not high, but constant, like a thermostat. Have your eyebrows professionally plucked. And grow your nails long (stubby nails, stubby girl). Exfoliate! See to cracked heels, cracked lips, grazes, bruises, calluses, rough skin, and hair in inopportune places. One excruciatingly stylish woman of my acquaintance has a single hair growing directly south from her otherwise pristine chin. It is possible she keeps it there for pure entertainment value, but, for me, that single hair quite ruins the undoubted power of her several Chanel jackets.

We all have our own beauty minefields, of course. Personally, I have learned to ignore my upper lip at my own peril. Given that sporting facial hair of any description is an unparalleled *faux pas* in the protocols of femininity, I have entered into an agreement with several girlfriends that if we ever end up incapacitated and unable to wield tweezers, we will visit each other at regular intervals to prune and bleach. This is staggering vanity, of course—but our fear is that without maintenance we could quite easily end up looking like Ben Stiller in *Dodgeball.* Our family and friends would flee the bedside in horror.

If similarly afflicted, you have a number of routes to redemption: You could wax, which makes you feel like a transsexual preparing for the Big Op. You could tweeze, which carries with it the old wives' tale that the chosen hair will return, bigger and stronger than before, like Popeye after a can of spinach. Or there's always electrolysis. I can assure you from experience that this is precisely as painful as poking yourself in the eye with a sharp stick. "There are more nerve endings per square inch here than on any other part of the body!" my therapist told me gaily as she inserted a very long needle into a follicle. "There's only a minimal chance of scarring!" she added, zapping like mad while my eyes streamed and my nose ran all over her French manicure. These days, I find bleaching is best.

My argument here is that seemingly insubstantial things can kill a look at a glance. The devil, as any fashion editor will tell you if you ask politely, is not in Prada. It's in the details. This is why a stylist rarely ventures out without a kit of canny essentials that will avert many a sartorial or cosmetic crisis. Your emergency rations should, at the very least, include old-time favorites such as safety pins, dressmaking pins, needle, and thread. At home, keep spare buttons handy, together with nipple concealers, stain-removal wipes, pumice, tweezers, and a lint brush. Carry a cotton ball or two for mascara spills, a tissue, a toothpick for spinach, and a small mirror (to check for spinach). And at home,

TAN YOURSELF THIN

By some fabulous trick of the light, a tan will shave off pounds, leaving you slender and toned without you even leaving your lounge chair. This is the fast-track to thin, but using the sun to do it is all wrong. A little lick of sun exposure is no bad thing (it is thought to combat depression and aid sleep); just don't overdo it. Instead of splaying yourself out in the midday sun, slathered in baby oil and reading John Grisham, go for one of the spectrum of tanning products on the market. Find out what works for you. It may be airbrushing, bronzing mist, sunless foam, tanning gel, tinting mousse, sun-kissed moisturizer with SPF and a free toothbrush. Just don't risk UV exposure (that's A *and* B, for those of you who aren't concentrating at the back). With any and all of these, the rule is to exfoliate first and wash your hands afterward. A gradual buildup will make you look less radioactive; don't go suddenly orange and surprise your friends by turning up at a barbecue looking like an Oompa-Loompa.

drape a silk scarf over your beautifully made-up face while you slip on your cashmere sweater. It's the least Elizabeth Taylor would have done in those heady old days.

76 GET A HAIRSTYLE THAT WORKS WITH *YOUR* FACE, NOT THE FACE OF THAT GIRL IN THE MAGAZINE

Wanting to resemble our heroines is nothing new—women have always dreamed of having Audrey Hepburn's smile or Marilyn Monroe's wiggle. But let this be a lesson to you: I once went to a hairdresser clutching a magazine photograph of Jennifer Aniston and her Rachel cut (it was a while ago). I returned to the office and my boss said, "Ooh, very Cyndi Lauper!" See? So many ways to fail.

According to celebrity hairdresser James Brown (the stylist who looks after Kate Moss), there are fat-busting ground rules for hair. "Don't follow trends," he says unequivocally. "Hairstyles are not shoes—they won't look great on everyone." And flatter your face: "A square jaw needs a choppy cut below the chin, whereas round faces tend to suit a shoulder-length cut with a few layers."

My own hairdresser, the redoubtable Jo Hansford in London (dubbed "the best colorist on the planet" by American *Vogue*), knows the healing power of a great cut and color. "It takes the attention off the body and onto the face," she says, offering these additional bits of advice.

* Make a round face longer by letting the hair grow to halfway down the neck.

* For long faces, try bangs with a jaw-length bob; that way, you're effectively cutting the length of the face in half.

* If your face is heart-shaped, loosely curl back the ends away from your face to add width at the chin.

And what about color? If you tend to have pink-toned skin and blush easily, Jo counsels caution. "Stay away from warm tones—the golds and reds—because they'll make you look flushed. Go for cooler ash-browns, wheat-blondes, neutrals, and caramels. And roots!" Yes? "White roots make the hair look thin, they make you feel old and bald. They stop you being the best you can. . . . " Which is, after all, what this entire book is about. So get your gray done; it's not only aging, it's disheartening. Personally, I always feel 3 pounds lighter when I leave Jo's salon with swishy, glossy, thoroughbred hair. (The feeling is fleeting, though, since my favorite restaurant happens to be next door. Curses.)

77 LEARN HOW TO GIVE GOOD PHOTO

Generally speaking, I'm okay to look at. Not pageant-winning, you understand. But decent. I don't frighten kittens, and on a good day I scrub up well enough to garner an occasional compliment. Why is it, then, that photographs always make me look like Fiona in *Shrek?* I've got one vacation photo in which I'm the spitting image of Andy Rooney, so much so that people have started to ask why he was with us in a Menorcan tapas bar last summer. As one photo-phobic woman told the *Times* recently, "From looking at our photographs, you'd think my husband was married to the *au pair.* If I died tomorrow, my children would hardly have a single photograph to remember me by."

A survey by Hewlett Packard has found that two-thirds of us are "deeply embarrassed" by many of our photos. I'm with the majority on this one. I go from half-beauty to half-beast at the merest hint of flash. I always seem to be lurking on the periphery of any shot, red eyes ablaze, shirt askew. I have countless snapshots where my nose—*just my nose*—has crept like a lone adventurer into the foreground, as if sniffing for attention. It has taken me years to work it out, but the truth is that, until fairly recently, I have been a hopeless subject. Someone only has to point a camera in my general direction and my face plays dead, my mouth forgets how to smile, my eyes glaze over, and the wind blows in from the east to make my blouse billow out into the shape of a Mongolian yurt. When new photos appear, I scan them urgently for me, me, me, and I'm invariably crushed that the darling little nautical dress I was wearing has made me look like Georgie Porgie, having recently consumed both his pudding and his pie. In a world where image is all, where the airbrush is king, and where I regularly have my photo taken doing interesting journalistic things, this is no party.

David Lewis, PhD, a body-image expert and author of *Loving and Loathing: The Enigma of Personal Attraction*, has an explanation for this vexing state of affairs. We all apparently have three types of self-image: our "real self" (how we believe ourselves to be), our "other self" (how we believe other people regard us), and our "ideal self" (the type of individual we most want to be). "Our degree of liking or disliking [photos] of ourselves depends on how closely they match not our real self, but our ideal self," he says. "A photo which, through careful lighting and camera angle, makes you appear closer to your ideal self will be treasured and preserved."[1]

Right then: how to seize one of these super-shots for yourself? Over the years, I have made a point of gathering tips from those in the know—the A-listers who are forever under the eye of the paparazzi lens, the models who only have to breathe to make the cover of *Vogue*, the photographers themselves who know precisely when to press the shutter and when to stop for coffee. If you're forever de-tagging on Facebook, take a look at what I've learned and what I will try to remember next time I'm on vacation (with or without Andy Rooney).

When photographed, try to:

✱ Turn slightly sideways, one foot forward à la Liz Hurley, weight on your back foot. Stylist Charlotte Stockdale counsels: "Stand three-quarters to the camera, shoulders back, and smile with a closed mouth."

✱ Lengthen your neck, and tilt your chin marginally down (think Linda Evangelista, not Yertle the Turtle). This tip ought to lessen a double chin. If it doesn't, try a turtleneck. Dropping your chin will also make your eyes appear bigger. I know—amazing, isn't it? This is the Diana Tilt, as you will recall from the Princess's many interviews.

✱ Hold your arms fractionally away from your body to minimize the appearance of lady wings. "You can," says a fashion director at *Vogue*, "create the illusion of slimmer arms by turning the arms outward, palms facing forward, by your sides, so that the outer arms are against your legs." It's possible that you will look like a supplicating martyr in this pose—which is slimming, yes, but suspect on the beach in Ibiza.

* Shoulders back, abs in (but don't *suck*—you'll look as though you've just been slapped in the gut).

* Look away from the camera just before the click, and then turn back. Ah, says your face, it's *you!* This trick will give your eyes a chance to look "live" and you a reasonable chance of looking human.

* Your tongue rests gently behind your teeth, not glued to the roof of your mouth.

* Perfect your picture smile. If your mouth won't relax and behave, do a Keira Knightley: Just put your lips together and blow gently. Christy Turlington was also adept at this soft pout. Clearly, it helps if you are unfeasibly beautiful, but we civilians can try it, too. Don't try too hard or it will go all Louis Armstrong on you.

* Use your handbag to disguise your baggy bits. Grace Kelly did precisely this on the cover of *Life* magazine in 1956, when she shielded her baby bump with her Hermès purse. So patrician! You can do it with a cardigan slung over your shoulder or a husband slung into the foreground. Grab a child or something similar and station it in front of knock-knees, varicose veins, ugly shoes, etc. (Though why you're wearing ugly shoes is beyond me. Haven't you read Chapter 7?)

* Place your gaze very slightly above the camera when the picture is taken. Jacqueline Kennedy apparently used this technique; it also helps reduce red-eye.

* Model Sophie Dahl, who is similarly expert at taking a flattering photo, says "Don't chatter—you'll have your mouth open in the pictures and you'll look like a freak." If you possess a particularly animated face, as I do, settle it, or you'll look like a gargoyle.

* Avoid white dresses—they'll make you bigger, flatter, fatter. Yes, even the bride. Quite why the Victorians obliged a woman to wear white on the most important day of her young life is beyond me. If concerned on your big day, perhaps use bridesmaids, ushers, and sundry floral

arrangements by way of disguise (see page 173). Also, an ivory or coffee tone is generally kinder than stark white.

＊ Don't squint into the sun. Wear shades, or look the other way.

＊ If You're Desperate #1: Play with your hair. Diane von Furstenberg has been doing this in photos for decades, and it takes years off her, making her look youthful and adorable, like a foal.

＊ If You're Desperate #2: Look back over your shoulder toward the camera. Why do you think they're always doing that in the J.Crew catalog?

＊ Find a photographer who loves you. Mario Testino, perhaps, whose life's work it is to make women look beautiful. If Mario is booked, at least find someone who cares enough to make sure there isn't a flagpole sprouting out of your head.

＊ Once you've found a photographer who loves you (hey, no pressure, but it would be great if it was your partner, for convenience if nothing else), you now need to give them the heads-up on lighting. It's a girl's best friend and a woman's redeeming savior. Aim for a flattering light to give a softening, wrinkle-smoothing effect, rather than a harsh light, which threatens to create nasty nose shadows or raccoon eyes. Play with the lighting, know where the sun is, and consider your background colors. It may be a bit much for a quick snap, but it is worth understanding a little about light if you want to give yourself the best possible chance of a decent portrait. After all, it's going to be on your mother's mantelpiece for decades to come.

＊ Get your photographer to tilt the camera upward a smidge for a more flattering angle: It will elongate your face and improve your proportions.

＊ Always remember that photographs don't tell the whole truth. They are not a mirror image, so you're bound to be thrown by an unfamiliar version of your own face. According to Linda Papadopoulos, PhD, a U.K.-based psychologist, "Photographs aren't very representative of what we look like in reality . . . [they're] just a record of one static moment. People are never completely still like they are in a

IF MAGAZINES CHEAT,
THEN YOU CAN, TOO

Remind yourself, as you say "cheese" and hope for the best, that the images that surround us are pure, unrestrained fantasy. As supermodel Christy Turlington explains, "Advertising is so manipulative. There's not one picture in magazines today that's not airbrushed. It's funny—when women see pictures of models in fashion magazines and say, 'I can never look like that,' what they don't realize is that no one can look that good without the help of a computer." Or, as Cindy Crawford sums up, "I think women see me on the cover of magazines and think that I never have a pimple or bags under my eyes. You have to realize that's after 2 hours of hair and makeup, plus retouching. Even I don't wake up looking like Cindy Crawford."

Lately, the kind of airbrushing and retouching usually reserved for top models (who, heaven knows, are the last women who need it) has become available to the masses. Snappy Snaps has an airbrushing service for customers who want to enhance their photos without all the bother of a beauty overhaul. You can brighten dark circles, lengthen legs, erase a belly roll, and whiten teeth, just like they do in the art departments of magazines. If you want a deeper clean, 399Retouch.com can give you a complete picture facelift, eliminating saggy jowls, bags under your eyes, and unsightly husbands. The only thing you can't do is cut and paste an Adonis in a thong to stand at your side. Actually, hang on a moment . . . you *can* have an Adonis! There you go: the world's perfect picture.

Alternatively, cut out the middle man and do it at the source. You can now buy digital cameras with a "slimming feature" that stretches your image, visually removing about 10 pounds in the process. (Get your hands on an HP Photosmart R967 to try it for yourself.) It's called "digital dieting." Useful for Internet brides.

photograph, and animation changes the way we look. In studies, people are often rated as significantly better-looking in person than in photographs, and that's because of personal qualities, such as confidence." This, I like.

* Finally, don't run scared of the camera or you'll end up with vast tracts of your life undocumented, the you of your youth lost forever. Besides,

DON'T GO FOR THE SELL; GO FOR THE CELLULITE

Laser energy, vacuum massage, micro-encapsulated caffeine tights, infrared light, guarana soap, jeans infused with retinol serum, radio frequency, crossed fingers, liposuction . . . the incredible choice of everyday miracles available to the poor woman afflicted with cellulite points out what a persistent and universal problem it is. In 2007, a full 85 percent of American women were encumbered with the stuff, which is a heck of a lot of women walking out of their bedrooms backwards. This vast expanse of orange peel is undoubtedly a serious worry for a serious number of women. Cellulite is, alas, predominantly a girl thing, its formation closely linked to female sex hormones, which is why, as a rule, men have no need for infrared pants.

As anyone who has it knows, cellulite is formed as fat cells enlarge with age. The bastards. They nudge up against connecting fibers, a bit like a balloon being blown up through a pair of fishnets (one of those delightful images we could really do without). What you see on the surface is a characteristic dimple effect, which sounds cute. Cellulite is not cute. It is a curse. So zap it. Stop thinking "wonder fix," and start thinking "I wonder if I can fix this?" Stop tinkering about with your exterior, and start work on your interior. I know it may not be quite as thrilling as buying a lovely bottle of goo in a pretty pink box, but the advice below will work—in time.

when you look at old photos that you once hated because you thought you looked fat and old and stupid . . . what do you see now? Not so bad after all, right?

* One more lighting tip: If you want sincere flattery, don't wait for your partner to come up with the goods. Do it yourself with votives. Or a jar candle. Or a collection of pillar candles installed on the coffee table as if

---

* **Eat well.** Embrace plenty of vegetables, fruit, and whole grains, while introducing a moratorium on processed food, sugar, alcohol, and caffeine. Some time ago, I remember reading the brilliantly titled *Cellulite My Arse!*, in which author Shonagh Walker recommended the consumption of foods that stimulate the detoxing process, such as celery, cucumber, leeks, and onion. Worth a try.

* **Hydrate.** Drink lots. Water, not coffee, not juice, not merlot. Good old H_2O.

* **Exercise.** To stimulate circulation, get up off your bottom. Show it to the world, not just your sofa.

* **Don't smoke.**

* **Slash salt.** It encourages fluid retention.

* **Go organic.** This will reduce your unintentional intake of estrogen and other hormones lurking in mass-produced meat.

* **Body brush.** Work upward with a dry natural-bristled body brush while humming to yourself. (Bathroom acoustics are always great, aren't they?)

* **Massage.** A lymphatic drainage massage may well help to stimulate that sluggish circulation. Even if it doesn't, it's a fine way to spend a lunch hour.

* **Self-tan.** Cellulite is much less obvious on darker skin.

waiting for a choirboy to sing "O for the Wings of a Dove." According to Adam Hall, director of photography for various films and commercials, "Candlelight is very warm, very soft, and irons out wrinkles and imperfections." Perfect, particularly for romantic assignations, cozy suppers, a girls' get-together. We're not, though, living in Dickensian London, so for everyday purposes, invest in superior lighting for your home. This is your space! It should work for you. Proper lighting—by which I mean plenty of choice from floor and table lamps with warm-colored shades, up-lights to bounce light off the walls, a hanging light with a wide shade pulled low over a dining table—will be so much kinder than an overhead strip, the kind of light that beats you up and leaves you for dead. Save that for your bathroom, where honesty trumps artifice every time.

78 TREAT BEAUTY PROMISES WITH CALCULATED CAUTION

There are certain bitter truths that the beauty industry and all its pretty messengers don't want you to uncover, partly because it would put them out of a job, but chiefly because it would forever pop the bubble of sweet-smelling hope that informs the whole expensive endeavor. So get with the program. Know, for instance, that models who look thin enough to have eating disorders usually have eating disorders. Know that time will indeed bestow fine lines upon your brow, and hypo-poxy-nutrino-placenta-extract in a costly porcelain jar will do little to help. Know, above all, that rubbing cream on your bottom will not shrink it.

Enticing as they seem, with their promises of smoothing, polishing, and melting away fat, cellulite creams are not going to do much more than exercise your credit card. Save your money—perhaps in that empty porcelain jar—and spend it on a rowing machine. Now, take a deep breath and wise up to your worst fears. Extract your head from beneath the blanket of deception and take a good look at your thighs. If there's cellulite there, get a grip and tackle it.

79 DO A DIANA AND GET A COLONIC

So, you're feeling baggy, gassy, and bloated? Your hair and skin are limp, and your tongue's an interesting shade of beige? It's alimentary, my dear reader. You ought to give some thought to your internal flora. I know it's not exactly dinner-party conversation (unless you're German), but what goes on down there can have a significant impact on how good you look in a bikini. Chew on the fact that our distinctly unnatural modern diet does our internal ecology few favors; overprocessed foods, high-fructose corn syrup, antibiotics, great slabs of meat . . . these things arrive in the gut and subtly upset the balance, like an ex at a wedding.

There are ways to improve your equilibrium. Bran, psyllium, and natural live yogurt are all good places to start. Heidi Klum recommends bathing in Epsom salts to reduce bloating; I recommend that you don't drink through a straw. If it's just a little local difficulty, the Gut Trust, which offers support to people with irritable bowel syndrome,

THE BEAUTY BREAKFAST

When you're weary, feeling small, what you really need is this energy-boosting, body-buffing breakfast. It promises to aid digestion and elimination, leaving you with beautiful, clear skin and bundles of get-up-and-go. Here's what to do.

* Before you go to bed, mix a tub of live yogurt with fruit juice or water to give it the consistency of a shake.

* Add a handful of old-fashioned oats, some seeds (sunflower seeds, flaxseeds), plus chopped prunes, chopped apricots, chopped dates, and chopped almonds.

* Put it in the fridge overnight to ferment.

* Eat it in the morning.

* Feel lovely.

recommends probiotics—those kindly bacteria that reside in small yogurt drinks or (better still) in acidophilus capsules—together with plenty of hydration.

If things really have seized up, you could always give colonic irrigation a whirl. You'd be in good company. Princess Diana made thrice-weekly pilgrimages to London's Hale Clinic where she underwent what fast became known as the Royal Flush. It was also a favored technique of John Lennon and of Mae West, who apparently started every day with a refreshing morning enema. "I'm sure," said her nutritionist Bernard Jensen, "that this simple practice greatly contributed to her unusual vitality, bright mindedness, and long-lasting attractiveness, as true beauty is but a reflection of the beauty within." Ah, true enough Bernard, true enough. Today, Kim Basinger, Goldie Hawn, and Demi Moore are said to be fans of irrigation, while Courtney Love swears by it. As she recently told *Harper's Bazaar* magazine: "It really did the trick for me . . . I hate reading magazines where the actresses are saying, 'Broccoli and fish, broccoli and fish.' You liars."

If you do decide to take the plunge, you'll find that a colonic *lavage* (as it is called in refined circles) is not nearly as dreadful as you might expect; I found it all far less embarrassing than I'd anticipated, a bit like childbirth or karaoke (though significantly less painful than both). Weight loss, though by no means its primary function, may be a welcome side effect.

80 LEARN TO USE BLUSH PROPERLY

I have a face shaped, broadly, like a plate. A generous observer might remark that it's more heart-shaped, but even a kindly soul would admit that I don't appear to have much in the way of cheekbones. I've always really fancied one of those wicked, chiseled faces that can stop traffic and fell men at a single stroke. Don't we all?

If you spend any time at all in the company of models, you'll soon notice that a potent alchemy goes on backstage at a photo shoot or fashion show. Prettyish girls with pasty faces, moon faces, pie faces turn up—and later (often much later), they emerge with the visage of Venus. They have been chiseled by Rodin, they are Muse, they are Grace, they are Siren. They have been lent high cheekbones and defined jawlines. They are slim of nose and long of neck. And it's all been achieved with the skillful application of cosmetics.

Clearly, most of us have more pressing engagements each day than walking to the end of a runway and back, ad infinitum or until someone lights us a Marlboro and tells us to stop—but many of the techniques known to the makeup gurus are well worth learning. They won't change your face completely, of course. You won't catch sight of yourself and think, "Ooh, hello Angelina!" But the judicious use of the principles of contouring will be yet another arrow in your quiver of weight-loss techniques, right up there with small plates and Magic Pants.

To get the lowdown (and the highlights) of contouring, I paid a visit to Terry Barber, a master in the art and creative director at MAC Cosmetics, the foremost international makeup brand for such endeavors.

Me: What is contouring?

TB: The art of contouring is the true art of makeup. Makeup itself was originally designed to accentuate the structure of a face rather than to decorate it. It's all about light, really. Darker colors will cause an area of the face to recede, while lighter colors will bring it out. You see the techniques most clearly on film and stage, but it's all about the trickery of makeup and it's something that can easily be adapted for everyday life if you know how. As a makeup artist, I've seen that what makes women really tick is when you give them a cheekbone, and better still if the method is undetectable. Eyes and lips come and go, they're trends, but makeup which enhances bone structure will be with us forever.

Me: Who taught you how to do it?

TB: I learned contouring from Liza Minnelli, who virtually worked in black and white. She'd put a little black under her jaw and cheekbone, and then blended it all the way up into the hairline, using the curl of her hair to accentuate the cheek. She would paint on a face, drawing on downward eyes—the "Halston Face"; she'd flick the contour up into the apple of the cheek and highlight the center of her chin and the T-bar of her face in white. It was pure showbiz.

Me: Anyone else?

TB: Yep. Linda Evangelista taught me a lot about contouring, too. She'd put a flick of dark brown under the chin to separate the face from the neck. But then, she lived on camera.

Me: Should we all be putting dark brown flicks on our chins? Wouldn't it look like a goatee?

TB: Products have changed so much lately, so it's much more subtle. I remember in the eighties, when it was all New Romantic, you'd have white skin and use gray to contour. You'd end up with stripes across your face. Now, though, pigments are jet-milled, really fine, with mineral formulas. These products "pop" the skin and don't look like a mask.

Me: Okay, so how do you do it?

TB: Here's how.

Shading: Contour products are meant to look like skin, so you see lots of taupes, beiges, ivories, flesh tones, darker skin tones—which can appear broadly similar to the untrained eye. Use a contour formula, such as MAC's Sculpt, to shade and give depth under a cheekbone, to narrow a temple or heart-shaped jawline. Go for a tobacco color that gives shade. But you don't want a dark brown jawline, so blend and play—always in good, even daylight if possible. Dust through the edge of the face.

Here's a foolproof trick for cheek contouring: Imagine a line (or hold a pencil) between the top of the ear and the corner of the lip. Shade that line. Imagine another line from the corner of the lip to the outer corner of the eye. Shading shouldn't come in further than that. If your face is wide, slim it down by applying contour color to the outer jawline; a darker shade below the jaw will make it more distinct. Like this . . .

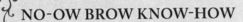

NO-OW BROW KNOW-HOW

You have the ultimate face shapers right there: your eyebrows. So get them to work on your behalf. I'm not expecting the full Janice Dickinson, but a little lift here, a lengthen there, can have a dramatic impact on a round face. Go pro if you can. If not, tweezers are your best weapon. Pluck after a shower, when your pores are warm and forgiving, and use a bright, inquisitive light. Get those stray midbrow hairs first, then pluck away *beneath* the brow, working toward a coquette's arch at a point that feels right for you. Terry Barber has the following tips: "Feather in the eyebrow with a pencil, using delicate strokes to elongate it by one or two hairs. The inner corners of the eyebrow shouldn't hook down too much—it makes the nose wider. Marilyn Monroe's sleepy glamor had a lot to do with those eyebrows. They were quite wide apart, with an arch directly above the pupil. It was all very architectural. . . . You can measure the ideal eyebrow by holding the pencil upright from the side of the nose to the brow. That's where your brows should start. Any closer and your nose will start to look wider."

Once you've plucked, brush your brows north with an old toothbrush, and trim unruly hairs with a small pair of scissors. If your eyebrows are scant, use powder eye shadow in the appropriate color to fill in the gaps, working in a light feathery motion. Very pale or gray brows may need tinting. If they are really sparse, an expert will be able to tattoo them in. (Go to the best salon you can afford; this is not an area for economy.) You can, of course, go too far with this. If you ever get to the stage where you are drawing on your own eyebrows in marmalade-colored pencil, you'll know it's time to put that mirror away.

Me: Oh, yes, that works! Should I use blush, too?

TB: Yes.

Me: How?

TB: The idea is to make your cheekbones look 3-D. Use a cream or gel blush and go up into the hairline. If you want, you can go beyond your usual contours to accentuate further than the natural shadow. Then you need to . . .

Highlight: Use ivory or a clear, shimmer product for accentuating the "crest" areas where light hits the face. Add a little cream highlight to the top of the cheekbone and the brow bone.

Eyes: Highlight from the inner corner of the eye socket to the bridge of the nose, right in that pocket of shadow. I call it "drawn-on surgery."

Nose: I wouldn't bother with nose contouring—it's a video technique. If you want to, just powder the sides of the nose to take off any shine (which widens the nose). We're talking about light, really, so leave the bridge of the nose unpowdered to give the illusion of narrowness.

Me: Brilliant. I have cheekbones! I have never had cheekbones. I think I might cry. (Etc.)

For similar hands-on advice, book a one-on-one session at a MAC counter. Ask for a member of the Pro team, who will have worked on fashion shoots and behind the scenes at runway shows; they'll know exactly how to release your thinner self.

9

MAKE A DATE WITH YOUR METABOLIC RATE

WHERE EXERCISE FITS IN

We all know the original fat-busting equation: To lose weight, you need to eat less or move more. It all comes down to the laws of thermodynamics. Fine—you can tinker around with pills and potions, ointments and self-help audio tapes. But if you want to succeed, you're going to need to stir yourself. Just a bit. Fairly often. The best way to get going is to introduce moderate cardiovascular exercise into your daily life. Don't book it into your diary as a special occasion; modify your lifestyle just a modicum and you'll see the difference next time you're stuck in a dressing room with only a 360-degree mirror for company.

81

GET BUSY. IT NOT ONLY BURNS CALORIES, BUILDS MUSCLE MASS, AND RAISES YOUR BASE METABOLIC RATE, IT WILL ALSO KEEP YOU OUT OF THE FRIDGE

A rather dispiriting survey by a skincare company not long ago found that we spend 14 hours and 28 minutes a day taking the weight off our feet—that's the equivalent of 36 years of our adult lives sitting down. Allowing for 8 hours of sleep, we spend a meager 1 hour 30 minutes on our feet, active, each day.

Yet we humans aren't programmed to sit, sit, sit. Physiologically speaking, we haven't changed a great deal from our days of roaming the great savanna in search of prey. We're designed to walk many miles a day, not cozy up to a computer screen with a box of chocolate chip cookies and a crick in the neck. So stand up, right now. Do something about it. Get in touch with your ancient self!

Exercise, if you're not already a fan, really needs to be something that you can weave into your life, not something you do as a grand gesture, expecting prizes and applause on your return. Do it in regular bursts rather than great blistering chunks.

The buzzword here is integrative exercise—which is a fancy way of saying "move around a bit more." Studies show that several 5- to 10-minute bouts of activity throughout the day will promote cardiovascular and respiratory health, lower your risk of diabetes, and improve your longevity. Start small: A brisk walk. A run down the road. A run back. Reach a new street light every day. Just don't expect a medal. (Unless you have just run a marathon, in which case, congratulations, it's all yours.) But watch out: Studies have shown that you're likely to pile up your plate if you've done even moderate exercise. So try not to see a run around the block as an excuse to eat four brownies as soon as you're back in the comfort of your own kitchen. Yes, you deserve a high-five, but not a high-calorie carb feast that leaves you with butter smeared on your chin.

Here, then, are a few tips on how to "thintegrate."

* **Use the stairs, #1.** Shun the elevator; cultivate claustrophobia; develop an unfounded fear of escalators. "Using the stairs is not seen as normal," says Amelia Lake, PhD, a research fellow in clinical medical science at Newcastle University. "In most [new] buildings it's very difficult to find a staircase. The focal point when you enter tends to be the [elevator]. In certain buildings, you'll even find that using the stairs will set off the fire alarm." Architect Will Alsop takes a stronger line: "If you really wanted to do something about [the obesity crisis]," he says, "You could take all the elevators out of all the buildings in London. Then people would be fit."[1] He's right. When employees of the University Hospital of Geneva were banned from using the elevator for 12 weeks—a move that increased their daily climb from 5 to 23 flights of stairs—their aerobic capacity increased by an average of 8.6 percent and their body fat levels fell by 2 percent.[2]

* **Find a way to enjoy walking more.** Fill your iPod with tunes. Hum. Snoop into people's front rooms, join the Neighborhood Watch, take up the lost art of perambulation in the park, perhaps while wearing a feathered hat. As you march, listen to stirring opera, or do as comedian Stephen Fry did and take your dynamic daily constitutional accompanied by a gripping audio-book: "You don't notice you're walking," reports Fry, "and you walk faster and faster because it's all very tense."

* **If you're into gadgets, get yourself a pedometer.** According to scientists at Stanford University, having a daily goal is an important predictor of increased physical activity. A review recently showed that pedometer use is associated with significant increases in physical activity and decreases in BMI and blood pressure.[3] Who cares if it makes you look nerdy? Better a fit nerd than a fat loser.

* **Discover pole dancing.** Consider belly dancing; take up tap . . . or just dance around the room. Whatever. Do it for 10 minutes a day, or every time you're waiting for water to boil. Choose your dance routine with care. If you take up swing, it'll cost you 372 calories an hour (especially if you do the East Coast Lindy Hop); belly dancing burns 378; salsa,

372; and ballroom burns 216 calories an hour (more if you do it in full makeup, silver stilettos, and a big swishy skirt).

* **Get off the bus one stop early.** Yes, I know you've heard it before, but have you ever done it? Do you even take the bus? If not, this one won't work for you. But if you do, run behind that bus and try to catch up, imagining that you have left your BlackBerry or your birth-control pills on the back seat. If you take the subway, come above ground at an earlier station and take in the view. Walk the rest of the way, looking upward to allow your gaze to rest on architecture you've never noticed before. Change your perspective.

* **Spring clean.** Commune with your inner control freak. Vacuum for 15 minutes and you've killed 58 calories.

* **Walk the kids to school.** Hey, it's better for them, too, so you're spreading the love. If you have no kids, walk someone else's kids to school (ask first).

* **Do one wild thing.** Abandon yourself. Get intense. Lose it on the dance floor.

* **Develop an interest in something arcane and hard to find . . .** like ammonites. Head out into the field (or to every museum you can get to) and find your holy grail.

* **Bid for a bike on eBay** and cycle to work.

* **Use the stairs, #2.** Instead of piling shoes and shampoo and Legos on the bottom stair so you can take everything upstairs in one trip, take things up one at a time.

* **Stand up!** Standing burns 36 more calories per hour than sitting does.

* **Indulge in impromptu games.** Play tag, hide-and-seek, basketball. You'll burn 100 calories in 10 minutes, and your kids will still want to talk to you when they hit puberty.

* **Consider getting a dog.** Energetic walking is known to be the single most valuable integrative exercise you can do, and an inquisitive terrier is as energetic a beast as walks the earth. I borrowed Rhubarb the Patterdale terrier from a friend a few months back, and my rather stagnant life was transformed as I was whizzed across the park each

morning. If you're single, a cool dog has the added bonus of being fantastic man-bait. Weimaraners and puppies work best.

* **Join a walking or hiking club,** or . . .
* **Indulge in speed shopping,** or . . .
* **Mail letters one at a time,** or . . .
* **Chi Walk.** This involves meditating as you walk, focusing on muscles and movement; its proponents promise that you'll get fitter—and slimmer—faster. You might also become a better person. Just think of the possibilities!
* **Drink more water.** You'll *have* to get up to go to the bathroom. Visit the one up three flights of stairs, not the one at the end of the corridor.
* **Lose the remote.** If elderly, keep forgetting where you left your teeth; if younger, make it your cell phone.
* **Move from the 'burbs.** A study of 200,000 Americans at Rutgers University in New Jersey found that city dwellers were on average 6 pounds lighter than their suburban counterparts, largely because, instead of driving, they walk more. "In very dense urban environments . . . there's an awful lot more walking involved, just because of the inconvenience of driving," said Tim Townshend, a former town planner quoted in the study.[4] Interestingly, city living creates what is known as the "eco-slob" effect, where the healthy, environmentally friendly option also happens to be the path of least resistance. By contrast, if your life is all mall and sprawl, you're more likely to travel by car and pack on the lard. This—together with the greater prevalence of gyms and lipo and bitchy girlfriends—explains why New Yorkers are slimmer than most other Americans.
* **If you are burb-bound, try "Mallercise."** This is the craze for power walking while window shopping. (Shoe manufacturers now market "mall walker" shoes featuring "extra traction for smoother, slicker mall floors.") On the plus side, mall walking is traffic-free, rain-indifferent, and relatively safe; it can burn 200 calories in 30 minutes, if you include the odd lunge and you laugh in the face of the escalator. On the down side, you may spot a must-have pair of ankle boots or a must-have Cinnabon. Either way, you lose the benefit.

82 FIND YOUR THING. STICK WITH IT. YOU MAY EVEN MEET AN ENDORPHIN

According to accepted wisdom, in order to lose 1 pound of fat, you must burn or dodge around 3,500 calories. Accepted wisdom can be so depressing, can't it? Well, fret not. Don't think lifetime, think lunchtime. Start now. A little jog. A step class for beginners. A cycle to work. Roller-disco. You choose.

If you have a wandering attention span and pathetic stamina (*moi aussi!*), you might need a goal. Before my wedding, for instance, plagued by the prospect of a small, backless white dress scattered with hand-sewn pearls, I somehow managed a session with a personal trainer three mornings a week for a year. And when I say mornings, I mean freakishly early—technically-still-yesterday early. We'd meet before 6, work out for an hour, and I'd be showered, dressed, and in the office by 7:15 a.m. Okay, so sometimes I didn't shower, but I *always* dressed.

Children change all that, of course. These days, I'm still up at the crack of dawn, but I spend those early hours searching high and low for a missing shoe or stirring oatmeal or trying to get orange juice out of the sofa cushions. In my more benevolent moments, I convince myself that all this rushing around is the rough equivalent of paying someone $45 an hour to put me through my paces on a cross trainer and then count while I perform 200 expert crunches. Not so. It's cheaper, yes, but nowhere near as effective.

Here is the bullet you need to bite: Proper exercise requires an element of planning, space-making, and commitment. You have to persevere. Tone was not built in a day. As an added incentive, it's worth noting that studies have found that the less muscle you possess, the harder it is to lose weight (because muscle is metabolically active, whereas body fat is inactive—as anyone furnished with a sizeable, sleepy rump well knows).

If you are obstinately vain, you'll also need to learn not to care what you look like when exercising. I'd like to say that I don't give a monkey's behind, but I've always found that exercising is a peculiarly intimate thing to do in public—a bit like speaking French or breast-feeding. I abhor sweating in front of strangers and will go to great lengths to avoid physical activity of any kind if it has to be done in a crowd. For this reason, my gym clothes really matter, perhaps more than any other outfit in my life. So I wear amazing stretchy, hold-you-in track pants by a yoga

MEET THE MIGHTY POWER ENDORPHINS

Exercise of any description is a potent mood-enhancer, as you'll notice if you compare the faces going into the gym with the ones coming out. Cardiovascular activity can escort you from the doldrums to the crest of a wave in a mere 20 minutes, its benefits being not only physiological but also psychological. You know you're doing yourself good, which is a real pat on the back; there's nothing like a well-used sneaker to put a spring in your step.

If you exercise in a concerted way for an extended period, you may even encounter the fabled glory that is an endorphin rush. Endorphins are produced by your pituitary gland and hypothalamus in response to strenuous exercise, excitement, or orgasm. They have a similar effect to that of opiates, in that they can relieve pain and bestow a pleasing sense of well-being and even euphoria.

Personally, I have felt many things during heavy exercise (hot, bothered, fatigued, angry, peevish, bored, a throbbing sensation in my left knee), but never euphoria. The conclusion I draw from this unscientific and selective study of myself is that I'm not exercising long or hard enough. If you do, however, it's possible that you too could experience a runner's high, and the point of enduring the undoubted hell of the New York City Marathon in the November cold will suddenly, blissfully, become known to you. More power to you, I say. Though the very existence of this exercise buzz has been questioned ever since the idea was first propagated in the seventies, German scientists have recently used PET scans and other technical wizardry to show that the limbic and prefrontal areas of a runner's brain (those associated with emotions) are indeed affected by the release of endorphins following a 2-hour run.

label called Prana. I like to think I look very slightly Cindy Crawford in dim light. (This is gym psychology, people, and it helps.)

The real poke in the eye is that most gyms are inhabited by a handful of jaw-dropping women who really *do* look like Cindy Crawford, even in very bright light. My advice is to ignore them. Ignore their bouncy pony-tails and their pert buttocks. Ignore their terry hot pants and their foxy tops. Concentrate on your mission. Hum if necessary. If time and commit-ment are issues, it pays to be choosy. Rather than go at it willy-nilly, decide which part of your body needs the most attention and target it.

* **Yoga** will give you a strong torso (from the abdominal work required to maintain those balancing postures) and muscular definition in your arms (if you stay long enough in Downward-Facing Dog). Muscles are lengthened through stretching, so regular yoga should leave you with a longer, leaner body. It also aids posture. Some forms of yoga are more dynamic and demanding than others. Regular Bikram or Ashtanga will clearly be more beneficial than lying down in a room that smells of patchouli while chanting "om" through your third eye.

* **Running** promises enhanced muscle definition and lower body fat, particularly if you go a long distance. Beware shin splints and jogger's nipple, also known as raver's nipple, weightlifter's nipple, and garden-er's nipple. (Though one suspects you'd have to garden freakishly hard to do any real damage.)

* **Walking,** like climbing stairs, should perk up your buttocks. "Walkers," fitness and diet expert Joanna Hall told the *Guardian*, "can have great buttocks as, unlike recreational jogging, with each stride the hip fully extends, targeting the gluteal muscles of the bottom, creating a firm, shapely, and uplifted posterior." Set a smart pace (see "How to Walk Off the Weight" on the opposite page), and keep those abs in. According to Hall, "the latest abdominal research suggests that training the abdominals in an upright position, as one ought to when walking with good technique, is more effective than traditional sit-ups as it builds the muscle in a func-tional way, doing something the body was designed to do."

* **Swimming** is a superlative all-around workout and will give you a defined waist and strong shoulders, together with toned pecs. If you're

blonde, it might also turn your hair green, so invest in a swim cap. And plantar warts are a constant threat. But don't let me put you off.

* **Pilates** will deftly streamline a body, the series of strengthening movements imbuing you with elegance, rather than hard-body tone. You'll

HOW TO WALK OFF THE WEIGHT

"Walking is potentially the most effective and accessible form of body-toning exercise," says fitness and diet expert Joanna Hall. "You can definitely walk fit, walk firm, and walk off weight. Technique and pace are crucial for best results. On my 28-day 'walk off weight' program [find out more at www.walkactive.co.uk], we have people walking off 10 pounds and 10 inches in just 4 weeks! Do it right and it definitely works."

Start by establishing your Optimum Walking Pace.

* Start to walk, progressively increasing your pace at 30-second intervals (speeding up your arm-swing really helps), until you are just about to break into a jog. This is your Break Point Walking Pace.

* Ease back off this pace by 5 to 10 percent, and you have your Optimum Walking Pace.

So no slouching, no foot dragging. No pigeon toes, no stopping for a cigarette or a muffin. If you're really going to walk your weight off, you need to do it with conviction (though that curious hip-rolling that long-distance competitive walkers engage in is probably a bit much). Settle for something that feels like an exercise rather than a stroll, with a quicker heartbeat and a bit of color in your cheeks. And, though walking in high heels is both an art and a sport, do wear properly fitted, springy sneakers if you want to walk fit. Doing it in Gucci slingbacks will do you no good at all. (Probably the only example of human endeavor in which this is the case.)

gain spine mobility and core strength, together with good alignment, which will make you an altogether more efficient beast, and all without breaking a sweat. Little wonder that an estimated 12 million people around the world practice it. Says Ron Fletcher, one of its devotees and teachers: "People mistake it for an exercise regimen, and it's not. It's an art and it's a science and it's a study of movement . . . you think about what you're doing." Using a reformer will isolate muscle groups for greater efficacy, though you may feel as though you're strapped to a medieval torture device.

83 WEAN YOURSELF OFF YOUR FAVORITE SHOW

We live in what experts call "an obesogenic environment"—a world that lends itself, inexorably, to the accretion of fat. For a quick overview of our fantastically busy, woefully lazy lives, consider the following snippets of data: The average American watches more than 151 hours of TV a month, but walks only 400 yards a day; 73 minutes of that same day are spent sitting in traffic; meanwhile, chores such as washing and cleaning are increasingly mechanized (electric toilet brush, anyone?). As a result, we are increasingly a donut-based life-form. And the striking thing about donuts? They don't move very fast.

If we'd care to admit it, most of us are prone to a pathological inertia. To do anything beyond breathing, sleeping, and snuffling through the contents of the fridge, we need a gentle push. Some of us may need a kick in the rump.

And the first hurdle is to switch off the box. Studies have shown that watching TV not only fosters inactivity and sloth, it also encourages mindless and repetitive snacking, inspired by the drumbeat of fast-food commercials. A University of Toronto nutritionist recently found that kids who watched TV while eating lunch consumed an extra *228 calories* compared to those who ate without the television on. "Eating while watching television overrides our ability to know when to stop eating," reported the Canadian Institutes of Health Research. In a similar study, the University of Michigan found that young children exposed to 2 or more hours of television a day were three times more likely to be overweight than kids watching fewer than 2 hours.[5]

Avoid Couch Potato Syndrome by keeping the TV in its place. In one room, not littered about the house on every available surface, as if you can't make it from the bathroom to the kitchen without finding out what's happening on *Lost*. Keep it mostly off. Turn it on when there's something specific to watch—it doesn't have to be an edifying documentary about life in Ancient Greece or how to install a composting toilet. But it could be something useful or uplifting or funny or piquant. Something memorable. You can really cut down on your TV time by deciding to stop watching—oh, I don't know—*Three and a Half Men*. Stop watching *My Mother was Built Like a Truck, Canine Masterchef, Honey I Ate the Kids*, or whatever the box is spewing out this evening. Stop watching addictive television—the sagas and soaps and series that sap your time and train you to need your nightly fix. Stop watching the eye-gouging pointlessness of reality TV shows, where you get to watch basic life-forms pluck their eyebrows and argue about corn-flakes. Snub the TV talent shows that suck you in with the promise that your phone vote will help decide someone's fate. Don't watch the foxtrot—learn it! It doesn't take a genius to recognize that settling down for another evening of glazed gazing into one corner of the living room, illuminated by the spectral blue of the screen, is a waste of everything except energy.

TV also tends to present a fantasy world of perfection, where anyone can be famous just so long as they can fit into a very small dress; this leaves the viewer feeling out-of-sorts and awfully susceptible to the pull of a cheering fatty snack. Oh, and if you do decide to watch TV, do it while you sit on an inflatable exercise ball. Do the same when you use your cell phone. May as well tone as you phone.

34 ALWAYS DO ONE MORE REP

The glory of exercise, no matter how half-heartedly you perform it, is that in time you get fitter. Things that made you retch with exhaustion one month can feel like a breeze the next—as long as you stick with it.

Don't think of it as a mountain to climb; it's not even a hill. It's more of a slight incline. Before long, you'll be at the summit, looking down on the poor suckers below who didn't stir their sorry selves when you did. Here's how to start.

❋ **Exercise early.** It's the most effective strategy for keeping new recruits on track; people who work out in the morning are 40 percent more likely to continue than those who postpone their workout until later in the day.

❋ **Tell people.** That way you'll stick with it. While men tend to be goal-oriented, women are gossip-oriented. A team from the University of Hertfordshire tracked more than 3,000 people attempting to achieve a range of things, including weight loss. They found that women were more successful at keeping their resolutions if they told family and friends about their plans, thus increasing their chances of sticking with the program by 10 percent. Share, go public, and you've nowhere to hide.

❋ **Incentivize.** This is one of my least-liked words, second only to "actioning." (Though "conversate" and "deliverables" put up a pretty strong fight.) But it does refer to a necessary requirement for the successful uptake and continuance of regular exercise: You need to feel like you are progressing. You need to be heading toward a goal, rather than meandering about in ever-decreasing circles until you lose the will to live. Incentives will help. Run to work for a month and spend the money you saved on gas or bus fare on a shiny new pair of shoes. Swim every day for a week and sleep in decadently late on the weekend, leaving the family to find the fridge on their own. Reese Witherspoon relies on the encouragement of Justin Timberlake and Coldplay; for you, it might be Rihanna or Prokofiev at full blast. Alternatively, try using bodybugg (bodybugg.com)—a device that tracks how many calories you burn, whether sitting at rest or exercising.

❋ **If motivation doesn't work, try coercion.** Put a contract out on yourself at stickK.com. The Web site—dreamed up by an economics professor at Yale—acts as a "commitment store" whereby you specify your goal and stake money on it. If you achieve the goal, the money comes back to you; if you fail, it goes to charity and you feel like a schmuck. Though it is largely dependent on self-regulation, you can add the frisson of peer pressure by having progress e-mails sent to family and friends, allowing your sister in Geneva to know if you've been lingering too long at the dessert cart. Dean Karlan, PhD, cofounder of stickK, explains that the Commitment Contract concept is based on two well-known principles of behavioral economics: "One, people don't always do what they claim they want to do; and two, incentives get people to do things."

* **Look the part.** I have taken to walking the children into school wearing my mildly snazzy gym clothes, all spandex and proper running shoes. This way, I arrive at the gates looking halfway decent, calm before the storm, and no one gets to see the "after" picture, when my face has turned a curious ruby red and sweat has puddled upon my upper lip. After a bracing run, I take the back route home and only ever meet one man and his dog. The dog casts pitying glances in my direction, but who cares? It's a dog.

* **Get real at the gym.** Of *course* everyone is looking at you. But they're also looking at everyone else. You may just hear tiny sighs of relief as people clock signs of cellulite, stretch marks, or rampant panty lines. The objective of the gym is to look great later, not while you're there.

* **Learn to love your sweat.** Take a tip from men, who have long known that there is status in sweat. But it has to be in the right place. At the gym, the wrong places include anywhere too close to your exercising neighbor, on back rests, and on handrails.

* **Talk-test yourself.** If you can comfortably hold a sustained conversation (or sing) during exercise, you're not working hard enough to gain aerobic benefit. Give your mouth a rest and work those glutes. If that all sounds too manic, relax. You really only need to . . .

35 KNOW THE POWER OF THE PUTTER

Scientists at the University of Missouri-Columbia have found that "puttering about" is just as valuable and effective an exercise as pounding

BURN BABY BURN:
CHART YOUR ENERGY EXPENDITURE

If you did a whole lot of nothing all day, lying in bed and dozing, your body would naturally burn roughly 1,400 calories. This is called the average base metabolic rate. It's just under a calorie a minute for an average-size woman (about 150 pounds). Irritatingly enough, men burn more—around 1,700 calories a day (or 1.2 calories per minute) if they are of average size (about 180 pounds). You can up the ante considerably by adding bursts of activity. For instance:

DO THIS	CALORIES BURNED*
Sprint for the bus	18
Browse shops for half an hour	68
Kiss in desultory fashion for 10 minutes	11
Play air guitar to whole of Lynyrd Skynyrd's "Free Bird"	250
Apply morning makeup for 10 minutes	33
Push a supermarket cart for half an hour	83
Vacuum the living room. Properly. Under the sofa, too.	58
Golf for half an hour	105
Clubbing, intensive	257
Perform karaoke, for instance The Carpenters' "Yesterday Once More"	10.1
The Beatles' "Let It Be"	11.4
Frank Sinatra's "My Way"	15.6
Guns n' Roses' "Sweet Child O' Mine"	21
Play Nintendo Wii, half an hour	75
Chew (sugarless) gum	11
Chew gum and fart at the same time	15.3
Fidgit for a bit	10

Figures are approximate and are in excess of normal resting metabolism.

*The number of calories required to run a kilometer is, handily enough, equivalent to your weight in kilograms—so a runner who weighs 71 kg will burn 71 calories/km. (To convert your weight in pounds to kilos, multiply it by .45) Isn't that neat?

away at the gym.[6] Ha! Ha ha! The research team discovered that many of the physiological changes in the body that arise between total inactivity and "puttering about" are more extreme than those between puttering and more strenuous exercise. What pleasant news. It may even call for mild celebration—a jig, perhaps, or a whoop of joy. Or a nice cup of tea with my friend Alfred, a man whose body barometer is set permanently to Putter Mode, a pace he has found to be perfect for the cultivation of runner beans, dahlias, and a general sense of bonhomie.

A further survey, this time of almost 20,000 Scots, found that just 20 minutes of moderate exercise, such as gardening or housework, *once a week* boosts one's mood—and daily physical activity is linked to lower stress levels all around.[7] So let's hear it for puttering—the ideal way to dispel crushing metaphysical angst!

While puttering like an engine at a traffic light is beneficial in so many ways, sadly the same does not apply to sitting on your tush. The researchers found that lipase, an enzyme that helps the body break down fat, is suppressed, almost to the point of shutting off, after a day without movement. When people sit—in front of a TV, a monitor, a computer game—fat is more likely to be stored as adipose tissue than to be passed to the muscles, where it can be burned. Sitting for prolonged periods thus results in the retention of fat, a lower level of HDL (that's the "good cholesterol"), and an overall reduction in the metabolic rate. Boo.

86 HAVE MORE ENERGETIC SEX. DO IT WITH THE LIGHTS ON

You probably think that everyone's at it. All the time. Banging away like Keith Moon. Coming like there's no tomorrow. Sex, more than any other human activity, is prey to Room B Syndrome—the feeling that there's a wild party going on next door and you're just not on the guest list. It's a fallacy, of course, promoted by unrealistic media chitchat and bogus "research" by companies that want to sell you innovative sex toys. But despair not. Recent figures show that on average, Americans make love between 4 and 10 times a month.[8]

The truth is, if we indulged even more often, we'd certainly be a fitter, saucier bunch. Beyond that, sex is well known to be a salve. It releases oxytocin, which begets intimacy and battles insomnia. It can improve self-esteem, combat stress, and also boost immunity to disease, linked as it is to higher levels of a natural antibody, immunoglobin A (IgA), which protects against colds and other infections. (Not exactly racy, I know. But interesting.) A half-hour romp

YES! YES! YES! HOW TO HAVE MORE SEX

* Before you love your partner, love yourself. You are gorgeous. Really. Chant this in the shower. Tell it to the mirror. And know that a woman who is embarrassed about the size of her backside is about as erotic as a flannel nightgown. Most men are grateful for all mercies, not just small ones.

* Get to know your cycle. The one in the hall, that is. Apparently, 20 minutes on an exercise bike can heighten a woman's sexual response. Cycling, in particular, improves circulation, which is the very crux of sexual function.

* Don't turn to food to turn you on. Dwell instead upon this anonymous thought: "Food has replaced sex in my life; now, I can't even get into my own pants." Let that be a lesson.

* But do eat well. Aphrodisiacs are, on the whole, worthless, though mildly entertaining on a long winter's night. According to Cambridge nutritionist Toni Steer, PhD, "Oysters are dead in the water: We know of no scientific evidence showing that any particular nutrients enhance sexual function or libido."[9] Bah. The best way to coax your libido up a notch is to eat a nutritionally balanced diet. I know, it's hardly rip-your-shirt-off sexy, is it? By way of consolation, some foods *do* support the natural production of

uses up 150 to 200 calories—about double the burn of golf, and easily twice the fun. If you do it in the "Italian Chandelier" sexual position, you will apparently consume up to 912 calories an hour. *Madre mia!*

Clearly, there's more than just fun and frolics at stake here: Tune in to your sex drive, and you'll look better. Look better, and you'll want more sex. See? It's one big circle o' love.

---

estrogen, which could help put a tingle in your jingle. These include pomegranate, fennel, and soy milk. (More on foods like these in Chapter 10.) Asparagus and avocados are high in vitamin E (considered to be a sex-hormone stimulant), while you may improve the bloodflow to your nether regions with the allicin in garlic. (Eat it, for God's sake—don't rub it on.) If you really want to get it on more often, ditch the triple-fudge ice cream (it makes a dreadful mess of the mattress) and serve Sex in a Bowl, instead:

WHAT

1 fennel bulb, thinly sliced
Juice of 1 orange
1 pomegranate (the excavated ruby seeds are really
    quite fetching)
A handful of young mint leaves, for color and bite
Chopped almonds for crunch (the aroma is also said
    to be a turn-on)

HOW

Mix together and serve.
Accessorize with a flute of Veuve Clicquot (optional)
Eat, kiss, get a room.

---

87 GIVE UP YOUR CAR

Use a carpool, instead. (Try a Web site such as carpoolworld.com or erideshare.com to find rides in your area.) Go on, live life in the fast lane! If your car is just too vital a component of your everyday existence—and I do understand how provocative it can be, sitting there in the driveway all shiny and capable—at least think about giving it a brief sabbatical. Hide your car keys the second Wednesday of each month. Never drive less than a half-mile (unless you are moving furniture or elderly relatives). Spill a skinny latte on the front passenger seat; you won't want to drive the thing until the smell has been dealt with by an expensive trip to a car detailer. (I have done this. It works.)

Really, it's worth reducing your reliance on the car for so many reasons—economical, ecological, ethical—but while you're dithering about and anticipating rain, chew on this: A study of 11,000 Atlanta residents reported a correlation between driving and weight gain. According to the findings, each additional hour spent in a car per day is associated with a 6 percent increase in the likelihood of obesity. So turn your life around: *Stop* driving to the shop that you can see from your own front door, *stop* driving to the gym, *stop* driving to lull your baby to sleep. Start to think before you drive.

88 SET YOURSELF A GOAL. RUN ON "HMPH" AND GO FOR IT

1. Enter a charity fundraising event—say, a swimming competition— and make your friends pledge money. You'll be too embarrassed to back out.

2. Sign up for a half marathon or the Breast Cancer 5k. How about climbing Mount Kilimanjaro or hiking the Grand Canyon? You think I'm joking?

3. Take a volunteer vacation. No more lounging by the pool with Sophie Kinsella or Danielle Steel. You could be building homes

FITNESS: NOT JUST IN THE MUSCLES, BUT IN THE MIND

Now, dear hearts, it's time to introduce you to one of my favorite pieces of research. It tops my list because it is pure and it is brilliant, and because it demonstrates a wildly provocative idea. The study, conducted by Harvard's psychology department, took 84 female hotel attendants from seven hotels, each of whom cleaned an average of 15 rooms a day. They walked and pushed and knelt and scrubbed. They carried and lifted and tucked and polished. But 66 percent of them reported not exercising regularly. More than 36 percent of the women said they got no exercise at all.

The researchers then divided the women into two groups, giving one set detailed information about the calorie burn of activities such as vacuuming rugs and cleaning toilets. They even put up notices in communal areas explaining the excellent health benefits of such work. After a month, the tutored group perceived that they did more exercise than before, while the untutored group's responses were unchanged. Neither group had altered their actual level of activity.

But here's the spooky bit: Despite no change in exercise level, the tutored group showed "improvement on every single one of the objective health measures recorded: weight, body fat, body mass index, waist-to-hip ratio, and blood pressure." The women in the informed group had lost an average of 2 pounds, lowered their blood pressure by almost 10 percent, and were significantly healthier than their uninformed sisters.[10]

It appears, then, that mind-set can influence metabolism. So tell me: What are you going to believe today?

in New Orleans with Habitat for Humanity, or helping to maintain the Appalachian Trail. It's all good, clean, energetic fun, and it comes with a made-to-measure halo. Find out more at habitat. org, responsibletravel.com, ecoteer.com, globalvolunteers.org, and americanhiking.org/volunteervacation.aspx.

4. Build something. A sailboat. A tree house. A den for the kids. A bookshelf. Make it something permanent, something that fills you with a righteous sense of pride. Try not to build Ikea furniture, which is impermanent and will fill you with a hideous sense of existential regret.

5. Enter a competition for which you are ill-equipped. Break dancing, perhaps, or kung fu. Aim to be a black belt by Christmas.

89 OH, AND SMILE MORE. LAUGH. IT USES UP ENERGY

There's plenty of evidence to support the claim that laughter is good for you. Apparently, as we chortle, muscles in the face and body stretch, blood pressure and pulse rise and fall, and we breathe faster, which transports more life-enhancing oxygen through the body. Research shows that laughter is also the best medicine: It strengthens the immune system, reduces food cravings (woo hoo!), and increases your threshold for pain. A real honking belly laugh burns calories; tightens up the abs, diaphragm, and shoulders; and, according to research presented at 2008's annual meeting of the American Physiological Society, reduces the amount of unruly cortisol coursing around your body.[11] A simple smile exercises 16 muscles in your face and increases the production of endorphins. Even a false smile can lift your mood. Try it.

Smiling more, looking on the bright side, walking on the sunny side—these will all help on a day beset by the blues. Find an exercise that makes you giggle. Take up badminton. Learn to roller-disco. Play Twister. If it feels good, you'll do it more often.

10

LIFE, THE UNIVERSE, AND EVERYTHING

⁓ ⁓

HOW ALL THAT YOU DO REFLECTS IN THE MIRROR

Your body, your diet, your health—none of these fascinating things exists in a vacuum. Now that you're within sight of the finish line, it's time to see that how you look, and, importantly, how you're perceived, is a function of a whole host of factors—some nebulous, some concrete. Your attitude. Your self-esteem. Your hormones. Your surroundings. Your agenda. All of these will dictate the shape you're in and how it feels to be there. Here's how to maximize your slimness potential by harnessing all the lifestyle quirks, the ways of living, that will turn your body around and deliver a great new you.

90 KEEP YOUR HORMONES HAPPY

As Tammy so rightly said, sometimes it's hard to be a woman. What she didn't say, though it would have been helpful, is that most of our problems don't have anything to do with men. They have to do with hormones. (I do appreciate that it wouldn't have made much of a song that way.)

You may not often dwell upon these ephemeral little doodads, but somewhere, everywhere, in the depths of your being, they control your metabolism, your destiny, your life; released by glands in the body, they have a multitude of overlapping, interweaving, fascinating functions, controlling all metabolic activities and basically calling the shots. We needn't go into the role of every blessed hormone here; what matters to us is that they affect calorie intake, nutrient uptake, and energy expenditure—the three factors that dictate the body shape you inhabit.

Countless studies have examined the role of hormones in weight loss and gain. Insulin, cortisol, adrenalin, estrogen, progesterone, DHEA—they all have an impact and it is in your best interests to find balance within to look better without. Losing fat is, after all, a biochemical process. It doesn't happen on the treadmill or at the fridge door. It happens in your cells.

Women are far more prone to fluctuating hormone levels than men are, so it really pays to keep your hormones happy by eating hormone-enhancing and balancing foods that will give you a better chance of staving off fat accumulation. According to Daniel Sister, a noted London doctor who specializes in hormone therapy, they will "help satisfy hunger, reduce cravings, stimulate the release of fat-burning hormones, improve the efficiency of your digestion, increase energy levels. . . . " They may even walk the dog, if you ask them nicely. The idea is to reject inferior fuel and start putting premium-grade gas in your tank. So:

* Increase your intake of vegetables, especially the cruciferous brassicas—kale, greens, broccoli, cabbage, cauliflower, and bok choy—all of which are particularly beneficial to your hormonal health.

* Soybeans will be similarly beneficial. Use soy milk instead of cow's on your morning cereal; drink miso soup as an instant warmer; choose tofu as protein once a week (more often, if it appeals; if tofu seems bland, choose the firm variety and marinate it in soy sauce, chile oil, ginger, garlic, and chopped shallot; or try the tangier smoked version).

* Sesame seeds, though small, are full of hormone-harmonizing goodness. Falafel with hummus, tahini, and shredded cabbage makes an excellent supper.

* Introduce more phytoestrogens (plant sources of estrogen) into your diet—such as sprouted alfalfa, chickpeas, cherries, parsley, licorice, flaxseed, rye, buckwheat, fenugreek, Korean ginseng . . . or, if this is all too complicated, simply turn to legumes, whole grains, root vegetables, and seeds. Or choose lentil soup. (You've been doing this since Step 11, so you're already ahead of the curve.)

* Avoid synthetic estrogens (used to fatten cattle and increase egg and milk production) by choosing organic. Your aim is for hormonal balance, so try to eliminate "estrogenic" substances from your environment. These pollutants, which can be found in plastics, hair dyes, and cosmetics, among other things, are capable of mimicking the effects of estrogen in the body. The symptoms of estrogen dominance include water retention, breast tenderness, PMS, mood swings, depression, loss of libido, heavy or irregular periods, fibroids, cravings for sweets and—you guessed it—weight gain.

* In fact, renounce PMS and all its evil, self-loathing works; vitamin B complex pills and evening primrose oil supplements should help mitigate its effects. You could follow the example of Gwyneth Paltrow, who was advised to consume brewer's yeast and eat more whole grains to get added vitamin B_6 into her diet.

* Include more essential fatty acids in your diet. So, more oily fish—mackerel, tuna, sardines, herring, and salmon—staying within recommended weekly guidelines. This is particularly important for women who have PMS, because the gamma-linoleic acid in omega oils can help iron out hormonal mood swings, leaving your vases and your

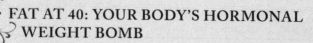

FAT AT 40: YOUR BODY'S HORMONAL WEIGHT BOMB

As Nora Ephron rightly warns in her book *I Feel Bad About My Neck*: "At the age of 55, you will get a saggy roll just above your waist even if you are painfully thin. This saggy roll will be especially visible from the back and will force you to re-evaluate half the clothes in your closet, especially the white shirts. . . . " This, alas, is something that happens to us all. It's even happening to Elizabeth Hurley. "The biggest change at 40 is that you can't stay slim with yoga or Pilates alone," she confessed recently. "You have to do something aerobic unless you don't eat much. But I eat lots. . . . "

When professional hard-bodies like Hurley are experiencing age-associated metabolism issues, you know something's up. As one wag put it, "The older you get, the tougher it is to lose weight, because by then your body and your fat are *really good friends.*"

The bitter truth is that everything flags in midlife. Dr. Daniel Sister says, "The first few pounds may mysteriously appear when you hit your mid-thirties—regardless of how much you eat or how much you exercise. Muscle tissue decreases and your body's basal metabolic rate begins to slow down. Your ability to burn calories is reduced, like a poorly burning chimney.

"A few years ago, research finally validated what we long ago suspected: fat cells have a gender. A woman's fat cells are physiologically different than a man's. They are larger, more active, and more resistant to dieting. As women enter their middle years, in response to lower [estrogen] levels, their 30–40 billion fat cells increase in size, number, and ability to store fat." The upshot, and crushing downside, of all of this is that menopausal women are highly efficient fat storers—and the belly is usually where everything goes to pot. All the more reason, then, to get in touch with your hormones and treat them with respect.

marriage intact. If you're a vegetarian, get added essential fatty acids from flax- or hemp-seed oil.

* Zinc-rich foods are hormone helpers. You'll find it in red meat, liver, nuts, dried fruit, and oysters.

* Exercise. It not only tones the body, increases muscle mass, releases anxiety, and maintains cardiovascular health and bone density, it also affects the hormone systems in the body. It does this by, among other things, increasing the responsiveness of cells to insulin and helping to metabolize cortisol and adrenalin, turning your body from one that stores fat into one that burns it. Retrieve those sneakers and start today.

91 AIM FOR LESS STRESS BECAUSE STRESS FEEDS FAT

Here's a surprise: Our demanding, challenging, competitive lifestyles have an enormous impact on our weight and shape. Rushed, stuffed eating; unpredictable mealtimes; low-grade nutrition—all of this has its pernicious effect, as evidenced in a study of 60 women at Yale University. Researchers found that, thanks to the release of cortisol, abdominal fat develops when a person is under long-term stress.[1] This hormone is produced during a fight-or-flight response, stimulating insulin release and promoting rapid fat and carb metabolism to cope with extreme demands. This serves to increase your appetite for high-starch, high-fat foods. So, if you are under constant stress—and nearly one in ten of us report that we are experiencing work-related stress to the extent that it is making us ill—cortisol levels are persistently elevated and, lo and behold, you always crave something deep-fried.

"There's good evidence to suggest that cortisol activates an enzyme which promotes fat storage in fat cells (adipocytes)," explains Joanne Lunn, PhD, nutrition scientist at the British Nutrition Foundation. "The number of receptors for cortisol is greater in intra-abdominal adipocytes, so the accumulation of fat at this site will be accentuated when levels of cortisol are high." In other words, stress turns women into apples. It also, adds Emma Stiles, nutritional scientist at the University of Westminster, "increases insulin and decreases female hormones," with all the waist thickening we already know this entails.

In a related study, researchers at the University of California found that stressed-out rats responded by drinking increasingly more sugar water and eating increasingly more lard. They got fat by cushioning themselves with "comfort" food. This, then, is why donuts always seem so consolatory and why Homer Simpson has them as a primary food group. ("Stressed" backward spells "desserts," as Homer himself might tell you.)

Oh, and to top it all like whipped cream on a sundae, stress also depletes all manner of beneficial nutrients—from the antioxidant vitamins (A, E, C, and vitamin B complex) to minerals such as zinc, selenium, calcium, magnesium, iron, potassium, sulfur, and molybdenum. Without those? Honey, you'd be nothing.

The goal here, then, is to let go a little. If you march through life with gritted teeth, heart palpitations, and a tense nervous headache, if you are certain that everything will fall apart if your pencils aren't lined up, it's time to engage in some stress management. Play squash, lift weights, meditate, spend time in a bubble bath and come up smelling of roses. If none of this helps, talk to a health professional.

92 SLEEP WELL

Are you sitting comfortably? Then let me introduce you to Leptin and Ghrelin. They may sound like characters from the *Lord of the Rings* trilogy, but these two are hormones, and here's what they do.

Leptin is the way your fat speaks to your brain. And what a profoundly fascinating conversation that must be. Leptin's role is to keep the hypothalamus informed about the adequacy of your energy stores; it's the satiety hormone. If the signal falters, the brain seeks a source of energy to fill the void. It boosts hunger and sends you off on a hunt for that chicken drumstick in the fridge. To make matters worse, a large fat cell, being large, produces a lot of leptin. When we diet, those fat cells shrink (the accumulated effect is what you marvel at in the mirror), and leptin levels fall. In a galling piece of negative feedback, this stimulates your hunger and encourages your body to conserve energy. Arrrgh.

Ghrelin, as we discovered earlier, is produced in the stomach to signal hunger to the brain; it's the hormonal version of a tummy rumble.

What, you may wonder, does this have to do with sleep? Well, leptin has a circadian rhythm and reaches its peak during sleep. If you're not sleeping well (and around one-third of us don't), peak leptin levels are not reached and the brain sends out its foot soldiers—hunger pangs and energy conservation—just as it does when your fat cells shrink during dieting. At the same time, lack of sleep causes ghrelin levels to rise. Your appetite peaks and the cookie jar calls.

There have been innumerable—sometimes controversial, sometimes hyperbolic—investigations into the effect of leptin and ghrelin on weight. These include:

* Stanford's study of 1,000 volunteers, which found that those who slept fewer than 8 hours a night had lower levels of leptin and higher levels of ghrelin, and (here's the rub) they also had higher levels of body fat. "Specifically, those who slept the fewest hours per night weighed the most."[2]

* A study at the University of Warwick found that sleep deprivation was associated with almost double the risk of being obese.[3]

* Researchers at Bristol University compared blood samples from insomniacs and good sleepers. The former had leptin levels 15 percent below normal and ghrelin levels 15 percent above normal.[4]

* A study at Laval University in Quebec found that there may be an ideal sleep zone of around 8 hours a night that facilitates body-weight regulation.[5]

* Jim Horne, PhD, professor at Loughborough University's renowned Sleep Research Centre, counsels caution in all of this, noting that "it seems that, at best, sleep plays a minor physiological role in causing obesity, although, there may be a more behavioral explanation, for example, via sleeplessness-induced lassitude and 'comfort eating.'"

Either way, what you need to absorb is that sleep is not just a passive zombie state; it is active, intricate, and vital to the smooth running of your metabolism. If we disrupt it with a 24-hour lifestyle, over-stimulating ourselves in the dead of night, working double shifts and long hours, eating at odd times, our bodies will inevitably suffer.

Whatever our hormones are up to, poor sleep will certainly rob us of the energy required to bounce out of bed and seize the day. This low-energy cycle is the arch-enemy of sustained weight loss, making us crave sugary snacks and caffeine pick-ups to get us through . . . which then serve to interrupt sleep patterns and so the whole sorry saga goes on and on.

HOW TO SLEEP EASY IN YOUR BED

According to the Sleep Council, two-thirds of people believe that they get less sleep now than they did a few years ago—around 90 minutes less, according to one leading U.S. sleep expert. "You probably have a generation that is quite sleep disturbed," agrees Kathleen McGrath, medical director of Sleep Matters, a helpline operated by the Medical Advisory Service. "I think we are looking at a time bomb. People now are not physically tired but mentally tired. . . . Some people's bedrooms look like the Starship Enterprise, lit up with TV screens and computers. Your bedroom is for two things: for sleep and for sex, not necessarily in that order."

If you toss and turn and clock-watch, your body is not getting the rest it so richly deserves. Jim Horne, PhD, professor at Lough-borough University's renowned Sleep Research Centre, has the following tips for restful sleep.

1. Pack up your troubles. Anxiety and overstimulation will interfere with sleep, so choose calm, relaxing activities before bed over watching TV, which is a stimulant. Dr. Horne recommends jigsaw

By now you should be feeling pretty sleepy. Great. Go to bed. Sweet dreams. (Not too sweet, mind you.)

93 STOP THINKING BIG AND TALKING BALONEY

Never utter phrases such as:

* **"I have a sweet tooth."** No, you are addicted to sugar. A note to all sucrophiles out there: Science has recently decreed that there is no

---

puzzles, walking the dog, knitting, and doing the dishes. Your kitchen will sparkle, and you might end up with a nice new scarf.

2. Rise at a regular time. No matter when you went to sleep, get up at the same time each day. This helps to program your body clock with a good sleep-wake pattern which, says Dr. Horne, can be hugely helpful for insomniacs.

3. You don't need 40 winks. Try 15. If you're feeling shattered by midafternoon, take only a short, 15-minute nap. Beyond that, and you'll eat into your body's sleep needs and disrupt your night.

4. Keep it cool. Your body needs to cool down during sleep. So no superheavy duvets, electric blankets, or central heating set on "Tropical." Nudge open the window, instead.

5. Go "shhh." Heavy curtains, eye masks, earplugs, blackout blinds. Do what it takes to avoid light and noise pollution.

6. Clock off. Melatonin can help reset the body clock, according to Dr. Daniel Sister. It's a hormone produced in the pineal gland to regulate sleep and wake cycles, but it can also be taken as a supplement (available over the counter) to help promote lovely lullaby sleep.

such thing as a "sweet tooth." Researchers at Duke University claim that the human brain senses that sweet foods are high in calories and "rewards" people by releasing hormones that make them feel happier.[6] It's not your tooth, sweetie, it's your brain. Train your brain, and junk the junk food.

* **"I have a big appetite."** Perhaps you do. But that's a confession, not an excuse.

* **"I have a slow metabolism."** So move around more!

* **"I am absolutely ravenous . . . I could eat my own liver! I am starving hungry . . . my blood sugar is dangerously low . . . if I don't eat that danish right now, I'm going to pass out!"** No, you're not. I'm guessing it's mere moments since your last meal. Get ahold of yourself, woman. If you find that your blood sugar suffers crazy spikes and dips, even it out by eating low glycemic index foods such as nuts, prunes, or whole wheat toast, not refined carbohydrates like muffins or cookies. These will simply add to the roller-coaster ride and send you over the edge in a hail of pie crumbs.

* **"Woo hoo! Broken cookies! That means all the calories have leaked out!"** This aphorism and others like it are not even faintly amusing. It is what greedy people say to successfully cross the bridge from one Milano to the next.

* **"I would rather be big and happy than on a diet and miserable."** I like the second clause of this sentence, but *big and happy?* More like fat and delusional. Don't diet, but *do* be honest with yourself.

* **"I have big bones."** Yup. And so does a woolly mammoth. What's your point?

* **"I was born fat."** Good grief. Where to start?

* **"It's just middle-age spread."** Trust me, that's the worst kind.

* **"I'm eating for two now."** If you are pregnant, all the more reason to stay healthy. Don't reach for the Twinkies as soon as the stick turns blue. You'll regret it all in about, oh, 40 weeks.

* **Stop starting sentences with "I always . . . "** Surprise yourself. I always do.

94 GET INTO THE GOOD LIFE AND GROW YOUR OWN VEGETABLES

Why? I'll give you 10 good reasons.

1. **Taste.** Home-grown carrots. Try them. You'll eat more. You'll see.

2. **Thrift.** Why pay $3 for a bag of arugula when you can grow it on the patio for a dime?

3. **Control.** You're in charge of what you spray on your lettuce. There's no multinational conglomerate breathing fumes all over them and shoveling on pesticide and then keeping them in a lock-up for months on end before they even meet a mouth. They are yours, all yours! Thus, unlike many a bag of store-bought, chlorine-washed salad, they're packed with weight-erasing vitamin-C vitality.

4. **Jamie Oliver.** He does it. Or at least someone does it for him.

5. **Eco-cred.** No packaging. No food miles. No guilt. Get into composting, and you're more ethical still. I would recommend a wormery, but, really, *eeeew.* In the *house?* I prefer to chuck organic waste into a composter, which manages to chow its way through eggshells, tea bags, all sorts of stuff—though not through silver teaspoons from the set you were given as a wedding present by Aunt Evelyn. That was a relief, I can tell you.

6. **Chill.** This is slow food—which, as we know already, makes it good food. It is necessarily local and seasonal. And it's relatively easy . . . so long as you remember to water your pumpkins, thin out your greens, pinch out runner beans, and mound the earth around your potatoes. Okay, so you may need a book. I recommend *Rodale's Ultimate Encyclopedia of Organic Gardening.*

7. **Exercise.** Weed the garden for 30 minutes and you'll motor through 150 calories. You'll probably need a manicure afterwards, too (so that's 50 more).

8. **Wellies.** Yes, these fashionable rain boots are the foundation of many a lovely outfit—particularly when paired with a rustic linen

apron, a gauzy floral dress, forget-me-nots entwined in your hair, that kind of thing. I'm all for homemade lemonade served in the garden on a warm day, perhaps with mismatched china and Aunt Evelyn's teaspoons. It's so rural chic. You'll look as though you've strolled nonchalantly from the pages of an Anthropologie or J.Crew catalog, smelling vaguely of rhubarb compote. Such joy, and a fashion triumph to boot.

9. **Camaraderie.** If you have never announced your arrival at a friend's house with a bag of home-grown potatoes, you've never lived. And in this economy, you may soon find an endless parade of acquaintances bringing boxes of fruits and veggies and homemade sloe gin to your door. This is a weight-loss dream—far better than arriving with a box of cupcakes.

10. **Boasting rights.** If you have a vegetable garden, you are a lucky minx indeed—forget an Hermès Birkin; what the fashionable really crave right now is a patch of tilled land upon which to sow microgreens. Seven million U.S. households are currently growing their own fruits, vegetables, herbs, or berries. Why not plant some tomatoes and zucchini in your backyard instead of the same old boring marigolds?

95 BECOME A BUDDHIST AND END DESIRE. OR FOLLOW THE TAO AND DO NOTHING

Now that we're nearing our destination on this journey to figure-happy bliss, it's worth asking yourself some philosophical questions. Do you always want more? Are you never satisfied? Are you sad and hungry? I only ask because these aching, yearning sentiments have come to typify life in the 21st century. I'm not about to get all "Confucius, he say" on your ass. But there is a lesson to be learned from the chronicles of ancient wisdom, and it will affect your relationship with everything in your world, including your lunch. The crux is to live consciously. With awareness. I know I sound like a fortune cookie, but this is important. It has to do with grand old pearls such as self-acceptance, responsibility, and purposeful living. If you have already switched off and switched on the

TV, just pause it. For a moment. Could you be kinder to yourself? Could you like yourself a little more? Could you tune into something a bit more constructive than the notch on your belt?

In truth, we all could. There's no need to get fanatical about this, mind you. According to idle rumor, Gwyneth Paltrow has in the past tried dining naked while sitting in the Lotus position in front of a mirror, in order to facilitate an increase in self-awareness. Clearly, this is something she undertakes in private, allowing the sight of her postprandial abdomen to put her off the leftover tiramisu in the fridge. You may find this somewhat difficult if you have guests over for supper. Better, perhaps, to concentrate on something more meaningful than your own belly button. As Cyril Connolly wrote in *The Unquiet Grave*, "The one way to get thin is to re-establish a purpose in life." And, had he thought about it, I'm sure he would have added that the purpose ought *not* to be "to have better buttocks" or "to get into a smaller bikini."

When you stop to think—and I urge you to, right now—most of us could do with connecting more and criticizing ourselves less. In this respect, I'm with Henry Miller, who said that "the aim of life is to live, and to live means to be aware, joyously, drunkenly, serenely, divinely aware."

We could, if we chose, live more in the present tense—here and now, not there and next. Interestingly, Buddha had plenty to say on the subject of body shape. "What we think, we become" was one of his. And, my own personal favorite when things are crap and the dress doesn't fit: "You can search throughout the entire universe for someone who is more deserving of your love and affection than you are yourself, and that person is not to be found anywhere. You yourself, as much as anybody in the entire universe, deserve your love and affection."

96 FIGURE OUT THAT FRIENDS CAN BE FAT MAGNETS

Just last week, I spent a lunch hour (more like 3 hours, but why quibble?) with my friends Pippa and Lou. We were in high spirits and all felt rather hedonistic and conspiratorial as we dipped great chunks of salty focaccia into a central pool of olive oil. We all decided to have

PUT A LITTLE LOVE ON YOUR FORK

Food really ought to be served with soul, love, and laughter, not peppered with caution, misgivings, and guilt. There's so much enjoyment in a shared snack, a special occasion cake, an innocent bowl of ice cream . . . really, thinking about it all too hard, weighing it up and worrying about the consequences simply sours the taste. Wouldn't it be better to rejoice?

By way of example, singing and eating always went hand in hand in our house when I was growing up. (Although it was well known that the pairing was considered rude in polite company.) Still, when sausages were popping in the pan or a roast chicken was sitting on its roost waiting to be carved, all manner of singing would break out. Mostly, we sang when doing the dishes, a nod to the well-known fact that singing makes a dull job go faster. My sister and I would do Abba, or hits from the musicals, with my mother doing her impromptu rendition of Nancy in *Oliver!*, all oom-pah-pah and Mr. Percy Snodgrass, while she wiped down the countertops. My father preferred snippets of opera sung to his own libretto. ("Toreador, don't spit upon the floor! Use the spittoon,

appetizers because, well, weren't we celebrating something? No? Oh well, why not?

Three large glasses of Chilean sauvignon blanc later, Pip had ordered risotto, Lou had the confit de canard, so—what the hell?—I ordered the linguine carbonara. I thought a side of fries would be good, just to share. It would barely be six fries each. We ordered dessert because no one was watching, and then we ate the chocolate mints that accompanied coffee, because . . . well, who could remember why? There might have been a second bottle of white. And suddenly, what do you know? We were *shopping*.

that's what it's for!" addressed to the sticky chicken glue from the roasting pan.) At Christmas, carols echoed around the steaming kitchen as the aunts and cousins, each clutching a damp tea towel, belted out "Good King Wenceslas" or "We Three Kings" and pirouetted across the floor in an attempt to avoid washing the heavy saucepans.

It was during one of these family get-togethers that I had a teenage wobble about what to wear out that evening to a disco. (Yes, it was that long ago.) My grandmother, a woman well versed in the value of golden dancing shoes, said in her no-nonsense way, "I wouldn't worry darling, nobody's going to be looking at you."

It has taken me years to realize that she meant it not unkindly, but as a call for me to be less *involved* with myself. Since then, I've discovered scientific studies that show that my grandmother was dead right: People aren't paying half as much attention to you as you think they are. Most of the time, they're bound up in an infinitely more fascinating subject: themselves. So here's the thing. Sing more. Worry less. Remember that the person on the dance floor who looks as though she's having the best time, probably is.

It's not that girlfriends mean to make you eat and shop with such cavalier abandon. It's just that *you* doing it condones *them* doing it which means *you* do it, and so the happy, fatty carousel goes round and round until you end up in a giggling heap on the floor.

Brian Wansink, PhD, in one of his many brilliant experiments, discovered recently that an especially good way to gain weight is to dine with other people. In *Mindless Eating: Why We Eat More Than We Think*, he reports that, "on average, those who eat with one other person eat about 35 percent more than they do when they are alone; members of a group of four eat about 75 percent more; those in groups of seven or

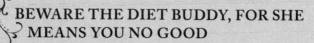

BEWARE THE DIET BUDDY, FOR SHE MEANS YOU NO GOOD

Diet buddies aren't always the faithful friends you need when you want to slim down. As a colleague of mine says, somewhat bleakly, losing weight is "like entering a war zone. There are no more friends. Keep in mind that no one really wants you to succeed." Personally, being of a more optimistic hue, I'd like to think that women have more solidarity than that—but even so, it's worth keeping your wits about you when you hear any of the following:

* "But I don't want to drink alone."

* "You don't need to lose weight!"

* "I cooked it especially for you because I know how much you like flourless chocolate cake with whipped cream *and* fudge sauce."

* "Oh, stay and finish the bottle."

* "I know you said you wanted a single scoop, but there was a special offer on this triple-banana split sundae with extra toffee sauce, chopped nuts, and those dear little mini marshmallows."

* "Have this last pancake; I'm just going to throw it out, otherwise."

You need to know that these are all the ploys of the saboteur. Tell her to back off or you'll start bringing your own grape seed extract to supper. More crucial, though, than avoiding the naysayers and the feeders is to do as you would be done by. As Balzac stated, "the more one judges, the less one loves." So stop appraising, stop weighing up your peers, stop competing, stop feeding your friends Boston cream pie in the hope that they'll burst free from their annoyingly flimsy little camisole tops. And start with a modicum of kindness, remembering that what goes around, comes around.

more eat 96 percent more. . . . If you want to lose lots of weight, look for a thin colleague to go to lunch with (and don't finish the food on her plate)."

In fact, it can work both ways, particularly among women. As a rule, we tend to calibrate our restaurant order with what other women at the table have chosen, the gluttony or abstinence of the occasion being precisely socially sanctioned. In my experience, and to corroborate Wansink's research, if the first bid is fairly high (a risotto primavera, say), the players will indeed go on to trump each other, adding side orders of buttered new potatoes and extra portions of hand-cut fries, until the final one to go finds herself in the embarrassing position of having ordered the entire left-hand side of the menu.

And yet, the whole game can play out differently. If Philippa starts off with "just a salad," Jodie will have the same, but with the dressing *on the side*. It all depends on the friends (underbidding is very popular in fashion circles), and the opening bid. Working logically, if a table of six fashion editors goes out for lunch, the last one to order could well go home hungry, possibly resorting to stealing the free mints from the bowl at the door to sustain her through the afternoon. (Yes, that was me.)

The more at ease you are, though, the more likely you are to indulge in piggery (which is why many of us gorge when eating alone). It's also why vacationing with friends is as dangerous as it gets; consider vacations the shark-infested waters of your social map. I recently went away with friends and the sheer quantity of food that was bought, discussed, consumed, and discussed again was phenomenal. Every third minute, someone seemed to be nudging another spoonful of mashed potato onto my plate. We'd eat and pick and chat and then eat some more, the constant ongoing conversation being about what we were going to have for the next meal and how many Mallomars were still left in the cupboard.

It's understandable, of course. Humans are social beasts. Eating brings us together. Food is brilliantly celebratory and cohesive, a lip-smacking, heartwarming social glue. You can well imagine that in those

WHY FAT FRIENDS ARE FATTENING

A study at the University of California recently showed that obesity spreads within social networks and that people with fat friends are 50 percent more likely to be overweight than those who hang out with skinny people.[7] Further research by economists at the University of Warwick, Dartmouth College, and the University of Leuven, found that people are powerfully but subconsciously influenced by the weight of those around them.[8] It turns out that "fattitudes" are contagious. It's all relative. If your friends and family regularly dig into a bucket of deep-fried chicken wings, you'll inevitably do the same. If they go for the hyper-Slurpee at the movies, your mega-Slurpee starts to look paltry by comparison. Says Professor Andrew Oswald at Warwick, "Rising obesity needs to be thought of as a sociological phenomenon, not a physiological one. People are influenced by relative comparisons, and norms have changed and are still changing."

long-ago caves, our ancestors sat around arguing about the relative merits of wild boar over raw bison—and not worrying a bit if they looked a little lardy in a loincloth. These days, though, if you are serious about keeping your figure under control, you need to find ways to be with friends without putting on a lot of weight—and without coming across as a supercilious bore who knows the calorie content of the table napkins. One good way to do it is to buy all of your girlfriends this book. Then you'll be on the same page, so to speak.

97 CHOOSE A CHALLENGE; DON'T GET TOO COZY

Okay, you can't move to another country or get engaged or divorced every time you feel your waistband get a bit tighter—but there is good evidence to suggest that a seismic shift in your lifestyle is what will really change your shape. Don't get contented, like a dairy cow. Don't settle, don't succumb, don't submit or slouch your way into an easy, acquiescent life.

"There is," said author Iris Murdoch, "no substitute for the comfort supplied by the utterly taken-for-granted relationship." And a glorious thing it is, too. But one of the greatest obstacles to weight-loss intentions is very often your partner, particularly if you have been in the relationship long enough to get thoroughly comfy, like a pair of old socks. If you're happy to burp in front of him, if you shave your legs while he shaves his chin, if you wash his boxers, then you are comfy. (If you iron them, you're insane.) But comfy is like a sofa: squashy, stationary, and quite hard to get out of.

Studies regularly show that women put on weight after they get married—partly because the prospect of that strapless organdie gown with cathedral train and accompanying bridesmaids is no longer blocking the view every time they look a cupcake in the face. But also because, once hitched, you tend to settle down, eat up, and order an extra portion of garlic bread. To coin an old proverb, as far as your figure is concerned, the most dangerous food is wedding cake. ("Matrimony," said one astute observer, "is a process by which a grocer acquires an account the florist had.")

Once married, it's all too easy to start eating big. Where once you'd have subsisted on a quick bowl of cereal for supper, now you're cooking a roast and all the trimmings. You didn't used to *do* trimmings. Now you're making gravy! As the *Observer Food Monthly* magazine notes, "Married people are feeders by nature. They do not fear carbohydrates, they get offended if you only eat half of everything. . . . Beware the following: bread on side plates! Mashed potatoes! Sauces! Married people love them."

Once children are on the scene, your parental lifestyle (if that's not too grand a term for it) probably means that you stay in a bit more and go out a bit less. Housebound, you're tied by some unseen umbilical cord to the cookie jar and the refrigerator. You down a glass of wine as soon as Olivia's little head hits the pillow, your reward for a day of motherly forbearance (and the fact that you managed to make an entire farmyard tableau from Play-Doh while doing three loads of laundry). Little wonder your prepregnancy jeans appear to come from another galaxy.

This isn't just idle observation. Weight Watchers recently produced a study of 3,000 married women that revealed the different stages a female figure goes through over the course of a lifetime. Almost 66 percent of those surveyed said their weight fluctuated depending on how happy they were at a specific time. According to the study, in the early days of a relationship, when a woman has found her dream man, she's "so keen to impress that she even orders salad for a romantic meal." Yikes. Next,

DEATH AND CHOCOLATE: HOW MORBID THOUGHTS BREED HUNGER PANGS

Sometimes, a piece of research comes along that allows you to stand back and marvel at the incomparable intricacy of the human condition. Here's just such a study: According to new research at Erasmus University Rotterdam, people who are thinking about their own deaths have an urge to consume more. A paper published in the *Journal of Consumer Research* reveals that "consumers, especially those with a lower self-esteem, might be more susceptible to over-consumption when faced with images of death during the news or their favorite crime-scene investigation shows." They explain this effect using a theory called "escape from self-awareness." When people are reminded of their inevitable mortality, they may start to feel uncomfortable about what they have achieved in their lives and whether they have made a significant mark on the universe. One way to deal with such an uncomfortable state is to escape from it, perhaps by having another generous handful of Jelly Bellies. The lesson here is to dwell not upon death, but on the life in you yet. (I did actually get that one from a fortune cookie.)

she enters the Comfy Zone, when cozy nights in with her fella, a DVD, and Chinese takeout mean she'll pile on an average of 11.3 pounds. As the Big Day approaches, our heroine loses (on average) 9.2 pounds to squeeze into the Big Dress. The first baby brings many delights, among them an average of 16 pounds of additional weight. Then, eventually, comes The Reinvention, when a woman realizes that there is more to life than sweatpants and daytime television. She drops more than 15 pounds, whoopee, just in time for perimenopause to sabotage her efforts.

How, then, to arrest the life-cycle lard? Your mission is to keep challenging yourself, stay out of ruts, shake up your life. If you always eat a huge meal with your partner, sign up for a dinnertime yoga class and make lunch your main meal of the day. If you find yourself doing the same things three evenings in a row, run to the end of the road and back as a penance. If your kids keep you in at night, take up piano or French or (better still) kickboxing. Get an instructional DVD: It will do you a lot more good than watching the entire five-season series of *The Wire*. Finally, once more from our old friend Honoré de Balzac: "Marriage," he wrote, "must constantly fight against a monster which devours everything: routine."

98 TAKE YOUR PASSIONS OFF THE PLATE AND INTO ACTIVISM. MARCH, NOT STARCH!

If the thought that gets you most excited in life is whether or not you'll fit into the next season's arrivals at Saks, then you need to recalibrate things a bit. Who knows where your energies could take you once you stop fretting and fussing about your own sweet self. Fund-raising? Raising bees? Overthrowing the state? It matters little what it is, but, with this wholesale overhaul of your life and behavior (look, you're at Number 98; there's no stopping you now), you should be in the market for refocusing your attentions away from the size of your rump and on to something that might make the world one speck better. If you're going to get intense, ardent, fervent—far better that the object of your attentions is something that really matters, such as your favorite charity, a local youth club, or a fundraiser for trees to be planted at the end of your street. (Go on, plant the trees yourself.) You'll be surprised by how much your body will benefit from a viewpoint that looks out, not in.

99 TAPE A PICTURE OF BAD BRITNEY TO YOUR FRIDGE. YOU WILL PUT DOWN THAT SLICE OF PIE

Britney's soul mate Madonna has this to say on the subject of body management: "If you want to know how I look like I do, it's diet, exercise, and being constantly careful." Constantly. Careful. Clearly, most of us inhabit the intermediate territory, lodged in a halfway house somewhere between Bad Britney and Meticulous Madge. But we all need regular nudges and prompts to remind us of the game plan, recognizing that saying No! to the pie has an immediate cost (no pie!) but—like flossing or pension plans—little immediate benefit. The benefit will come, with luck and a continued effort, tomorrow and tomorrow and tomorrow. To remind yourself of this, leave the wedding invitation on the mantelpiece, the cocktail dress hanging on the back of the bedroom door, the bikini shot taped to the tub of vanilla in the freezer. It's well worth keeping one eye on the calendar, too; there's nothing like a pool party in July to put you off that second sausage. A series of social deadlines will stay your hand as it wanders off in search of superfluous sustenance.

The idea here is to know your foe and keep it at bay using a combination of vigilance and exquisite *sangfroid*.

100 IN EXTREMIS, KNIT

You don't only eat when you're hungry. Eating can be a response to stress, fatigue, loneliness, euphoria, or grief. In particular, though, we eat when we're bored. Research has shown that half of adults do exactly this, reaching for a bag of Doritos or a handful of Cheez-Its simply because they'll occupy another small slot in the endless loop of your existence. It's a robotic, repetitive response to the featureless tract of time between here and there. It's why most of us eat a ton of chips and chocolate on a long car trip, and why a coffee break at work seems to make the day go

BOREDOM EATING: DO SOMETHING MORE INTERESTING, INSTEAD

* When a food craving strikes, Hollywood actresses are said to reach for their knitting needles rather than a giant bag of pretzels. Julia Roberts and Uma Thurman both do it, and you can't move backstage at fashion shows without getting jabbed by crochet hooks and cable stitch needles. You can charm yourself with the knowledge that knitting is incredibly cool, thanks to a recent resurgence among celebrities, anarchists, and guerrilla-knitting groups such as Cast Off and Knitta (a gang that "tags" statues around the world with subversive bits of knitting). You could even join a knitting circle. The winter nights will fly by, and you'll end up with an interesting sweater rather than an empty bag of Kettle Chips and a hollow void in your soul. Check out knitty.com for ideas.

* Chew gum. To paraphrase Lyndon B. Johnson, "like Gerald Ford, you can't eat and chew gum at the same time."

* Give yourself a manicure—it'll take care of your hands till lunchtime. The same goes for watercolors, scrapbooking, and bassoon lessons. Make your own Christmas cards, pet your cat, sew an enormous quilt from scraps of discarded clothes and then auction it for charity. I really don't care what you do, as long as it's not mindless mastication.

faster (especially if accompanied by a muffin). Food, though, is not the solution—it's the fuel. It's meant to take you somewhere, not leave you stranded on the sofa wondering where the day has gone. If you find comfort and solace in the ridges of a Ruffles potato chip, you really need to get out more. Find another crutch.

11

LOVE THYSELF

TALK YOURSELF UP
TO SLIM YOURSELF DOWN

After almost 20 years in the style business I have come to one clear
conclusion: How you look has, in truth, very little to do with your
weight. But it owes everything to your confidence. Think about the
women you admire, the ones who've got it and know exactly what to do
with it. I'll bet a pair of my very best Jimmy Choos that they exude
confidence, spirit, and verve. Building your confidence will breed a
healthier relationship with food and a better relationship with your
body. This is what you came for. This is what you've got—an intimate,
intuitive awareness that you are wonderful. You don't need your bathroom scale to tell you this. You know it, deep down, beneath the slimming embrace of that sensational dress you're wearing.

ACCENTUATE YOUR POSITIVES; TALK YOURSELF UP; RADIATE

Not long ago, I came across the word "numinescence." I have clasped it to my heart ever since and treasured it like the jewel that it is, despite the fact that somebody probably made it up—perhaps while watching a sunrise or drinking their third bottle of wine. A dictionary will tell you that the word "numinous" can be applied to something that is "awe inspiring" or "sublime," from the Latin *numen*, meaning deity. Numinescence, though, is more of a hybrid, a marriage of numen and luminescence. I like to think of it as "*It*," a quality that's intangible, timeless, and transcendental; it's the thing that,

NOT A DIET BUT A DO-IT: HOW TO CAPTURE CONFIDENCE

* **Get on your own team.** If you're not in your own cheering section, then why should anyone else be? It's just a basic tenet of good psychiatry. You've got to be positive, yelling "You can do it!" into the very center of your soul.

* **Know that you are not alone.** A recent survey found that 72 percent of women rated their looks as "average" (this is, you'll notice, a statistical impossibility). Interestingly, women who were more satisfied with their own beauty were significantly more likely to think that nonphysical factors—including happiness, confidence, dignity, humor, intelligence, and wisdom—contribute to making a woman beautiful. Look, no woman on earth loves everything about her body; so find the bits you do. Use this book to help pinpoint them. Cherish them, own them, rely upon them.

* **Know what's normal.** You need to understand that a normal woman, a good woman, can be soft and round. Look at Liv Tyler, a startling beauty who refuses to succumb to Hollywood stan-

if you could bottle it, would turn you into an instant billionaire.

Just try to stick *It* in a bottle, though, and the whole lot would spoil. Being volatile and personal, it can't be bagged, labeled, and shipped around the globe to be shoved on a shelf in Barneys or Bloomies, no matter who tries. Numinescence, then, is the butterfly that cannot be caught, the gossamer glow of mystery, nuance, and energy. You don't buy it with a credit card; you buy it with confidence. Confidence and love.

Consider Botox, by way of example. Why do women who have injected their faces with botulism always look so sour, so desperate, ironed of all glory? My feeling is that it's because they're afraid to inhabit their own faces. This collapse in confidence shows, even through the

---

dards: "To the rest of the world I am slim," she says, "and I like the way I am."

* **Aim for progress, not perfection.** Perfect is excruciatingly dull. It is your fallibility that people will fall for.

* **Know who's incredible.** Yep, you are. As Nigella Lawson once quipped, "Like I say to Charles [Saatchi, her husband], I don't ask for much, just 100 percent adoration all of the time. That's not so unreasonable, is it?" Not to me, it's not.

* **But do stay alert.** As your body becomes toned and slimmer, sister beware. Success breeds complacency and complacency breeds slackness, which breeds a chirpy little voice inside your head saying that one pudding pop couldn't possibly hurt. You're right. But three in a row is a recipe for disaster.

* **Be constant.** Staying slim does require willpower; no one is going to do it for you. It's your body, your life, your fudge brownie with hot chocolate sauce, fresh whipped cream, and choice of two toppings. Or not.

* **Be happy.** It will keep you in better shape than being hungry will, trust me.

---

taut shine of their skin. By contrast, think of women who know and enjoy themselves. You don't encounter many, not in an age devoted to undermining our self-belief and selling us a fantasy in disposable packaging. But when you do, when you're in the presence of numinescence, it is memorable and affecting, your whirring mind trying to place what it was about that woman—Her perfume? Her smile?—that made her stay with you long after she'd left the room.

There are, of course, famous women who have it in their very soul. Cate Blanchett. Julia Roberts. Selma Hayek. Julianne Moore has it. So does Oprah. Helen Mirren's got it. Elizabeth Taylor would have been lost without it. Catherine Zeta-Jones appears to have been born with it, the fuel for her incandescent trajectory from a humble town in Wales to Hollywood high society. But you needn't be a celebrity, or unconscionably thin or rich, to find your center and revolve around it.

Take Rose, a woman I met once at a party some years ago. I've written about her before, but she's well worth revisiting, like an old friend. We were in Lewes, feasting on honeyed Madeleines and local wine—and there, among the eclectic mix of guests (a woodsman from a nearby field, a girl with interesting teeth who made organic burgers from her own beef herd, a professional cyclist in yellow Lycra), there was Rose. She was perhaps 60 or thereabouts, with the kind of hair that simply won't behave in public, the color of steel wool and cut in a nothing-to-speak-of way. She wore no makeup and was broadly as beautiful or as ugly as the next person along. And yet, Rose shone. What was it? No Botox. No microdermabrasion. No cutting-edge designer clothes. We talked about this and that—a new house, an old joke—while my quizzical eye roamed about to exact the source of her magnetism.

What dawned on me later is that Rose was at one with herself, with her body, her age, her style, her shape. The effect of all this ease was startling. She wore those funky floppy layers that work so well when you're done with the fizzy little explosions of fashion. Rose coupled a charcoal-gray base of skirt and loose shirt with a stunning necklace of silver and amber, heavy with its own history, a necklace with a story to tell, and a capacious shawl of embroidered fabric in claret and tan, which she shrugged closer to her shoulders as the light faded and the temperature dropped in the backyard. The shawl might at one time have draped across an East Indian bed, or hung on a wall; it was ethnic, like patchouli, but rare, like gold.

For a seasoned old fashion hack like me, moments of epiphany are, surprisingly, rarer than gold. They were a dime a dozen when I first started at the catwalk-side, wowed by the sheer force of a Gianni Versace show or by Linda Evangelista's legs or by the unutterable perfection of a Dior gown. But through all that, the most potent images of style for me have come from people who understand not the current axioms of fashion, the gossip on the street, the nervous attachment to today's cult handbag or the must-have shoe. They come from people who understand themselves.

This, then, is numinescence—a make-believe word for an intangible thing. I've encountered it elsewhere, too. In my first yoga teacher, for instance, a glorious woman who wore only white and managed to maintain enviable equilibrium and body balance, despite a run-in with breast cancer and subsequent mastectomy. Or my friend Iris, who wears, mostly, wellies and a vast old sweater upon which (I believe) her golden retriever once had puppies. She's the kind of woman who finds daisies in her hair and wears corduroy. She's out of synch, but Iris manages the madness by being uncommonly content in her own skin. I envy her in a way I never would a woman in possession of the latest Prada bag (and believe me, I *love* Prada bags). Or there's the top-rung fashion editor who sailed through the bitch and bustle of the international collections, true always to herself and her style (a series of sober, sophisticated dresses in neutral tones, a wardrobe of perfect shoes), as if she nursed her very own secret, perhaps supplied at a crossroads in return for her soul. I remember watching her out of the corner of my eye as she'd sit at the catwalk-side, serene and captivating, while fellow editors squawked and preened, jittery in their Beau Brummel collars, their must-have jackets and monogrammed shoes. While they looked desperate to be someone—anyone—else, she looked nonchalantly happy just to be herself.

So how to capture a bit of *It* for yourself? By now, you'll have read and absorbed 100 ways to help you make a start. You'll know that the very act of dieting will inevitably make you feel cruelly dissatisfied with who you are, and that the drip-drip of the diet industry is pure poison, leaving you prone to quick-fix extremism and vulnerable to the snake-oil merchant and the triumph of hopeless optimism over experience.

Losing weight, then, isn't only about the ins and outs of your feeding habits. It's about you and how you feel about yourself. Start with self-acceptance. Start, if you dare, with self-love. It will give you a far more positive and dynamic platform for change, and you won't bore yourself into a hole with the constant drone of self-doubt. As Eleanor Roosevelt had it in one of her oft-quoted epigrams, "No one can make you feel inferior without your consent."

"When we are at peace with ourselves," says psychologist and weight expert Kerry Halliday, PhD, "the body finds its own natural weight. Searching outside ourselves for happiness is one of the reasons we fall prey to the quick fix. Eating problems are often the consequence of a disassociation of self from body. So become physical. Dance. Lighten up. Love yourself again." You don't have to be a rampant narcissist, but you could give yourself a break. You could stop rewarding yourself with food. You could start today. Couldn't you?

ENDNOTES

꧁ ꧂

Chapter 1

1 Hayley Dohnt and Marika Tiggemann, "Peer Influences on Body Dissatisfaction and Dieting Awareness in Young Girls," *British Journal of Developmental Psychology* 23, no. 1 (2005).

2 Ben Fletcher, Karen J. Pine, Zoe Woodbridge, and Avril Nash, "How Visual Images of Chocolate Affect the Craving and Guilt of Female Dieters," *Appetite* 48, no. 2 (2007).

3 Suzanne Higgs, PhD, A. C. Williamson, and A. S. Attwood, "Recall of Recent Lunch and Its Effect on Subsequent Snack Intake," *Physiology & Behavior* 94 (2008).

4 Kevin Devlin, "Thinking Yourself Thinner Is Possible," *Daily Telegraph*, April 23, 2008.

Chapter 2

1 Hamid R. Farshchi, "Beneficial Metabolic Effects of Regular Meal Frequency on Dietary Thermogenesis, Insulin Sensitivity, and Fasting Lipid Profiles in Healthy Obese Women," *American Journal of Clinical Nutrition* (January 2005).

2 Wayne W. Campbell, "Eating More Protein in the Morning Helps Dieters Retain Fullness," *British Journal of Nutrition* (September 2008).

3   Jim Waterhouse, "Chronobiology and Meal Times," *British Journal of Nutrition* 77, no. 1 (April 1997).

4   Bonnie Beezhold and Carol Johnston, "The Impact of Vitamin C Depletion on a Short-term Diet," presented at the Experimental Biology presentation in San Francisco, 2006 (part of the scientific program of the American Society for Nutrition).

5   Calories from meals versus snacks, figures from the U.S. Department of Agriculture's "Continuing Survey of Food Intakes by Individuals," 1994–96, 1998.

6   According to Information Resources Inc, the food industry research firm, as reported in the *New York Times,* July 7, 2007.

7   Rita Coelho do Vale, Rik Pieters, and Marcel Zeelenberg, "Flying under the Radar: Perverse Package Size Effects on Consumption Self Regulation," *Journal of Consumer Research* 35 (2008).

8   Brian Wansink and Junyong Kim, "Bad Popcorn in Big Buckets: Portion Size Can Influence Intake as Much as Taste," *Journal of Nutrition Education and Behavior* 37, no. 5 (September 2005).

9   See http://www.fsascience.net/2007/12/27/dump_the_detox.

10 Timothy W. Jones, "Using Applied Anthropology to Understand Food Loss in the American Food System," *Biocycle,* May 1, 2005.

11 William Clower, *The Fat Fallacy: The French Diet Secrets to Permanent Weight Loss* (New York: Three Rivers Press, 2003).

12 Heather Niemeier, "Internal Disinhibition Predicts Weight Regain Following Weight Loss and Weight Loss Maintenance," *Obesity* 15, no. 10 (2007).

13 Saima Malik, et al. "Ghrelin Modulates Brain Activity in Areas That Control Appetitive Behavior," *Cell Metabolism* 7 (May 2008).

14 Michael Boschmann, "Drinking Water May Speed Weight Loss," *The Journal of Clinical Endocrinology and Metabolism* (January 2004).

15 Heinz Valtin, "'Drink at least eight glasses of water a day.' Really? Is there scientific evidence for '8 x 8'?" *American Journal of Physiology* 283, no. 25 (2002).

16 Glass of water study at University of Washington, reported in Integrated and Alternative Medicine Clinical Highlights, August 4, 2002.

Chapter 3

1 Ana Marie Cox, "If Your Bra Doesn't Fit, Go Shopping," *Time,* June 27, 2006.

2 P. G. Wodehouse, *Very Good, Jeeves!* (London: Penguin Books, 1930).

3 See note 1.

Chapter 4

1 Maria Conceicao de Oliveira, "Impact of Fruit Intake on Weight Loss," *Nutrition* (April 2003).

2 Michael Zemel and Rachel Novotny, "Calcium for Weight Loss?" *Obesity Research* (April 2004).

3 Barbara Rolls and Julie Flood, "Eating Soup Will Help Cut Calories at Meals," presented at the Experimental Biology Conference in Washington, D.C., May 2007.

4 "Consumption of Soup and Nutritional Intake in French Adults: Consequences for Nutritional Status," Institut Scientifique et Technique de la Nutrition et de l'Alimentation, Conservatoire National des Arts et Métiers, Paris, April 2001.

5 Japanese meat-eating research from "United States Leads World Meat Stampede," Worldwatch Institute, July 2, 1998.

6 Stephen Nohlgren and Stephanie Garry, "Benefits may outweigh risk in fish dinner," *St. Petersburg Times,* March 9, 2008.

7 Megan Goldin, "Garlic, the Wonder Drug?" *Reuters,* December 3, 2001.

8 James Hollis and Rick Mattes, "Effect of Chronic Almond Consumption on Body Weight of Healthy Humans," *British Journal of Nutrition* (September 2007).

9 C. L. Hsu and G. C. Yen, "Effects of Capsaicin on Induction of Apoptosis and Inhibition of Adipogenesis in 3T3-L1 Cells," *Journal of Agricultural and Food Chemistry* 55, no. 5 (2007).

10 N. Vogels, M. T. Nijs, and M. S. Westerterp-Plantenga, "The Effect of Grape-Seed Extract on 24-hour Energy Intake in Humans," *European Journal of Clinical Nutrition* (August 2004); Rafael de Cabo and David A.

Sinclair, "Resveratrol Improves Health and Survival of Mice on a High-Calorie Diet," *Nature* (November 2006).

CHAPTER 5

1 Beth Newcomb and Cindy Istook, "A Case for the Revision of U.S. Sizing Standards," *Journal of Textile and Apparel, Technology and Management* 4, no. 1 (2004).

2 Suzanne Loker, Susan Ashdown, and Katherine Schoenfelder, "Size Specific Analysis of Body Scan Data to Improve Apparel Fit," *Journal of Textile and Apparel* (Spring 2005); reference to Kurt Salmon Associates survey, 2003.

See also Marina Alexander, Lenda Jo Connell, Ann Beth Presley, "Clothing Fit Preferences of Young Female Adult Consumers," *International Journal of Clothing Science and Technology* 17 (2005).

CHAPTER 6

1 Lawrence Cheskin, "Lack of Energy Compensation Over Four Days when White Button Mushrooms are Substituted for Beef," *Appetite* (September 2008).

2 Tom Leonard, "Cafeteria Trays Disappear in U.S. Bid to Tackle Obesity," *Daily Telegraph,* August 26, 2008.

3 Brian Wansink, "The Office Candy Dish: Proximity's Influence on Estimated and Actual Consumption," *International Journal of Obesity* (January 2006).

4 Paul Rozin, "Smaller Food Portions May Explain the 'French Paradox' of Rich Foods and a Svelte Population," *Psychological Science* (September 2003).

5 Harold Goldstein, "Potential Impact on Menu Labeling of Fast Foods in California," (August 2008).

6 Brian Wansink, James E. Painter, and Jill North, "Bottomless Bowls: Why Visual Cues of Portion Size May Influence Intake," *Obesity Research* 13, no.1 (2005).

7   Lucy Mangan, "On a Roll," *The Guardian,* July 18, 2005.

8   Susan E. Swithers and Terry L. Davidson, "A Pavlovian Approach to the Problem of Obesity," *International Journal of Obesity* (June 2004).

9   Susan E. Swithers and Terry L. Davidson, "A Role for Sweet Taste: Calorie Predictive Relations in Energy Regulation by Rats," *Behavioral Neuroscience* 122 (2008).

10 Kathryn M. Sharpe, Richard Staelin, and Joel Huber, "Using Extremeness Aversion to Fight Obesity: Policy Implications of Context Dependent Demand," *Journal of Consumer Research* (October 2008).

11 Maggie Stanfield, *Trans Fat: The Time Bomb in Your Food* (London: Souvenir Press, 2008).

12 See note 11.

13 Quote from "Devil's Advocate: The World's Most Notorious Lawyer Defends Himself, *The Independent,* July 3, 2008.

14 Fran Abrams, "Piling on the Pounds? Blame 'Calorie Creep'," *The Guardian,* November 10, 2007.

15 Shopping psychology studies by Siemon Scamell-Katz of research consultancy TNS Magasin, May 18, 2009.

16 Pierre Chandon and Brian Wansink, "The Biasing Health Halos of Fast-Food Restaurant Health Claims: Lower Calorie Estimates and Higher Side-Dish Consumption Intentions," *Journal of Consumer Research* 34, no. 3 (2007).

CHAPTER 7

1   "Vertical Stripes," presented by Peter Thompson, University of York, to the British Association for the Advancement of Science in Liverpool, September 2008.

2   "Black Experiment," presented by Peter Thompson, University of York, to the British Association for the Advancement of Science in Liverpool, September 2008.

Chapter 8

1 Leah Hardy, "Why Do Women Hate Photographs of Themselves?" *The Times*, July 26, 2008.

Chapter 9

1 Paul Arendt, "Can Architecture Make You Fat?" *The Guardian*, January 3, 2007.

2 Philippe Meyer, "The Geneva Stair Study," the University Hospital of Geneva, September 2008.

3 Dena M. Bravata, "Using Pedometers to Increase Physical Activity and Improve Health: A Systematic Review," *Journal of the American Medical Association* (November 2007).

4 John Pucher, "Does Auto-Dependency Make Us Fat?" *American Journal of Public Health* 93, no. 9 (September 2003).

5 Harvey Anderson, "What Television Can Tell us about Childhood Obesity," *Canadian Institutes for Health Research* (July 2008); Julie C. Lumeng, "Television Exposure and Overweight Risk in Preschoolers," *Archives of Pediatrics & Adolescent Medicine* (April 2006).

6 Marc T. Hamilton, "Role of Low Energy Expenditure and Sitting in Obesity, Metabolic Syndrome, Type 2 Diabetes, and Cardiovascular Disease," *Diabetes* (September 2007).

7 Mark Hamer, Emmanual Stamatakis, and Andrew Steptoe, "Dose Response Relationship between Physical Activity and Mental Health: The Scottish Health Survey," *British Journal of Sports Medicine* (April 2008).

8 2005 Durex Global Sex Survey.

9 Lucy Atkins, "Five Ways to Boost Your Sex Life," *The Guardian*, January 16, 2007.

10 Alia Crum and Ellen Langer, "Mind-Set Matters: Exercise and the Placebo Effect," *Psychological Science* (February 2007).

11 Lee Berk, Stanley A. Tan, et al. "Cortisol and Catecholamine Stress Hormone Descrease Is Associated with the Behavior of Perceptual Anticipation of Mirthful Laughter," presented at the American Physiological Society, April 7, 2008.

Chapter 10

1 Elissa S. Epel, "Stress May Cause Excess Abdominal Fat in Otherwise Slender Women," *Psychosomatic Medicine* (September/October 2000).

2 Shahrad Taheri, Emmanuel Mignot, et al. "Short Sleep Duration is Associated with Reduced Leptin, Elevated Ghrelin, and Increased Body Mass Index," *Public Library of Science* (December 2004).

3 Francesco Cappuccio, "Meta-Analysis of Short Sleep Duration and Obesity in Children and Adults," *Sleep* (May 2008).

4 Shahrad Taheri, et al. "The Mechanisms for the Interaction Between Sleep and Metabolism," University of British, Bristol Neuroscience, December 10, 2004.

5 Jean-Philippe Chaput, "Short Sleep Duration is Associated with Reduced Leptin Levels and Increased Adiposity: Results from the Québec Family Study," *Obesity* (January 2007).

6 Ivan de Araujo, "Food Reward in the Absence of Taste Receptor Signaling," *Neuron* (March 2008).

7 Nicholas Christakis and James Fowler, "Obesity Spreads through Social Networks," *New England Journal of Medicine* (July 2007).

8 Andrew Oswald, "Imitative Obesity and Relative Utility," presented at the National Bureau of Economic Research conference, Cambridge Massachusetts, July 2008.

ACKNOWLEDGMENTS

My thanks to Lizzy Kremer, a woman of great insight who truly knows the value of a shared dessert.

Thanks also to David Forrer and Kim Witherspoon at Inkwell Management, and to the team at Rodale, who turned my trousers into pants and my fringes into bangs.

Finally, always, to Lily, Ned and Paul, the loves of my life.

INDEX

Boots, 154–55
Boredom eating, 227
Botox, 231
Boy shorts underwear, 54
Bras, 50–51, 52, 53
Breads, 116
Breakfast, 24–26, 179
Break Point Walking Pace, 193
Broke-Smith, Jean, 58
Brown food, 29, 116
Buffets, 121
Business lunch, 119
Butter, 87

Caffeinated beverages, 119. See also
    Coffee; Soda
Caffeine, 117
Calcium, 68–69
Calories
    in alcohol, 145
    in caffeinated beverages, 119
    exercise for burning, 190, 198
    food low in, 116–18
Canapes, 132
Capri pants, 98
Car, decreasing time in, 202
Carbohydrates, 27–29
Carbonated beverages, 130–31
Carpooling, 202
Carrot sticks, 116
Celebrity magazines, realistic perspective
    on, 10–11, 13–15
Cellulite, 176–77
Ceviche, 72–73
Cheeses, 117
Chicken, 116
Children and lifestyle, 223–24
Chi walk, 189
Chocolate, 86–87, 117, 124
Chokers, 159
Cholesterol levels, 199
Christmas time, eating and drinking during, 134
Cigarettes, avoiding, 177
Clothing
    accessories with, 159, 161–62
    age-appropriate, 113–14
    to avoid, 105–8, 107
    belts, 157, 159
    black, 96–98, 97, 159, 163–64
    body shape and, 99
    bras, 50–51, 52, 53
    buying, 98, 100, 103, 108–9

corsets, 60–61
    dresses, 89–93, 92, 157
    exercise, 197
    fabrics, 160
    feng shui, 110–13
    fitted, 95–96
    jeans, 93–95, 97–98
    lingerie, 55–58, 56–57
    loose, 95–96
    midriff and, covering, 165–66
    monochrome, 18
    necklines, 158
    opaque tights, 61–62
    optical illusions and, 158–60
    panties, 53–55, 62–64
    pants
        black, 96–98, 97, 163–64
        denim, 93–95, 97–98
        hem of, 97
        high-rise, 156–58
        optical illusions and, 159
    pockets in, 160
    prints, low-key, 164–65
    shoes, 150–51, 152–55
    sizes, 100–103, 102
    stores, 98, 100, 103, 108–9
    striped, 161
    swimsuits, 104–5
    tricks versus dieting, 88, 149
    vanity sizing of, 100–103
    waistline and, 156–58, 156–57
    women designers of, finding, 109–10
Cocktail parties, eating and drinking at, 132
Cod, grilled, 79
Coffee, 117
Colonic procedures, 179–80
Confidence, 48, 230–31
Connolly, Cyril, 217
Contouring makeup, 181–82, 184
Cooking, 36–37, 121, 124
Cooking shows, 142
Cooking spray, 117
Corsets, 60–61
Cosmetics, applying, 181–82, 184
Cravings
    dieting and, 7
    favorite fattening food and, 122–23
    managing, 227
Crawford, Cindy, 175
Crisp, Quentin, 18
Cross, Marcia, 13
Crudites, 116
Cusack, John, 29
Cycling, 188